Diagnosing DSM-IV Psychiatric Disorders in Primary Care Settings

An Interview Guide for the Nonpsychiatrist Physician

Mark Zimmerman, M.D.

*Associate Professor of Psychiatry and Human Behavior
Brown University
Director, Primary Care Psychiatry Research Program
Rhode Island Hospital
Providence, Rhode Island*

Psych **P**roducts **P**ress
East Greenwich, RI

Copyright © 1994 by Mark Zimmerman, M.D.
ALL RIGHTS RESERVED
No part of this book may be reproduced in any form or by any means, including photocopying, or utilized by any information storage and retrieval system without prior written permission from the author, P.O. Box 228, East Greenwich, RI 02818

DSM and DSM-IV are registered trademarks of the American Psychiatric Association. Use of DSM-IV in the title of this publication does not imply either review of or endorsement of the contents by the Association.

Printed in the United States of America.

ISBN: 0-9633821-4-4

To Caryn, Kyle, and Cali
For your understanding, support, and the joy you bring.

TABLE OF CONTENTS

Introduction 2
The 5 Minute Psychiatric Screening Interview 4
Major Psychiatric Disorders - Axis I
    Anorexia Nervosa 8
    Bulimia Nervosa 10
    Alcohol Abuse/Dependence 12
    Drug Abuse/Dependence 16
    Schizophrenia and Other Psychotic Disorders ... 22
    Assessing Delusions and Hallucinations 26
    Mania/Hypomania 30
    Major Depression 34
    Dysthymic Disorder 38
    Panic Disorder 40
    Agoraphobia 42
    Social Phobia 44
    Specific Phobia (Simple Phobia) 46
    Generalized Anxiety Disorder 48
    Posttraumatic Stress Disorder 50
    Acute Stress Disorder 54
    Obsessive-Compulsive Disorder 58
    Somatization Disorder 61
    Hypochondriasis 64
    Body Dysmorphic Disorder 66
    Trichotillomania 67
Childhood Disorders
    Attention-Deficit/Hyperactivity Disorder 68
    Conduct Disorder 74
    Oppositional Defiant Disorder 78
    Separation Anxiety Disorder 81
Depression and Anxiety Due to Drugs, Medications, and Medical Illness 85
    Medications Associated with Depression 86
    Medical Illnesses Associated with Depression ... 87
    Medical Illnesses and Medications Associated with Anxiety 88
Mini-Mental State Exam (Folstein) 89
Brief Psychosocial History 92
Current Psychosocial Functioning 94

INTRODUCTION

This book is a guide to assist the nonpsychiatrist physician in evaluating psychiatric disorders in primary care settings. Primary care physicians see more patients with psychiatric disorders, and prescribe more psychotropic medications, than do psychiatrists. Nevertheless, many research reports during the past decade have demonstrated high rates of underdiagnosis and undertreatment of mood, anxiety, and substance use disorders in primary care settings. In part, this may be the result of inadequate training in the recognition and diagnosis of psychiatric disorders. Most primary care physicians' sole psychiatric training was during their 6-8 week clerkship in their third year of medical school. These clerkship experiences are usually based in psychiatric hospitals or on locked psychiatric units in general hospitals; thus, the type of psychopathology seen during the clerkship bears little resemblance to the type of pathology seen in outpatient medical settings.

DSM-IV lists the disorders and their criteria, but it does not guide the user in inquiry for them. The *Interview Guide* consists of questions for the most common DSM-IV Axis I diagnoses. This book is not a standardized interview, to be started on page *x* and followed until page *xx*. Rather it is a quick reference to be used in the context of a clinical interview. If a patient complains of depression, the interviewer can turn to the section on major depression and assess the relevant symptoms. If there is a suggestion of excessive drug or alcohol use, the interviewer can refer to the long list of questions for diagnosing drug and alcohol abuse/dependence.

The *Interview Guide* contains 7 sections. First, there is a 5 minute psychiatric screening interview which represents a mental health review of systems. Sections 2 and 3 include questions to assess the most common Axis I adult and childhood disorders. Medical illnesses and drugs that frequently mimic or cause symptoms of anxiety and depression are listed in section 4. The fifth section is the mini-mental state exam which is useful in screening for cognitive defects and dementia, and the final two sections include a brief psychosocial interview and a current psychosocial functioning assessment.

The book is organized by diagnosis. Listed in the box at the beginning of each section are the DSM-IV diagnostic rules--which and how many criteria must be present (inclusion criteria) and absent (exclusion criteria) for the diagnosis to be made.

The exception to the diagnosis-based organization of the guide is for five psychotic disorders--schizophrenia, delusional disorder, schizoaffective disorder, schizophreniform disorder, and brief psychotic disorder.

Questions to assess delusions and hallucinations are given in one section, and differential diagnosis is outlined and discussed.

The guide should be used in conjunction with the DSM-IV manual or Mini-D. For most diagnoses covered in the guide, the DSM-IV criteria (or a slight abbreviation of them) precede the relevant questions. However, the criteria are not included in the five psychotic disorders in the "Schizophrenia and Other Psychotic Disorders" section. Moreover, the DSM-IV manual includes lucid discussions of differential diagnosis.

Most criteria are assessed by several questions, and follow-ups to the initial questions are preceded by phrases typed in bold face such as **IF YES** or **IF NO**. This is a shorthand way of instructing the interviewer to ask additional questions. For example, **IF YES** means that the ensuing questions should be asked only if the response to the preceding one was yes.

Use of this guide does not guarantee competence. Interviewing involves more than the recitation of listed questions. With experience the clinician develops a style that generates a database for making diagnoses, as well as beginning a therapeutic relationship. Psychiatric diagnosis is not just based on responses to questions. It also relies on observation and evaluation of affect, behavior, and cognition (the ABC of the mental status examination). Also, organic causes of symptoms must be ruled out. However, it is difficult to conduct a psychiatric interview if you do not know what questions to ask. That is the primary purpose of this guide.

Acknowledgement -- Semistructured diagnostic interviews have been widely used in psychiatric research during the past 15 years. I have been involved in developing some of these measures, and have been trained in others. The questions in this volume derive, in part, from this experience. Because there are only a limited number of ways to ask about such symptoms as appetite change, sleep disturbance, etc. the questions will resemble the questions from these interviews, and they deserve acknowledgement. Specifically, had not the Renard Diagnostic Interview, Diagnostic Interview Schedule, Schedule for Affective Disorders and Schizophrenia (SADS), Kiddie SADS, and Structured Clinical Interview for DSM-III-R not existed, then the present guide would not have been as rich and complete. The *Interview Guide* is more user friendly than these other research instruments because of its modular based approach to assessment that follows a brief screening interview. Moreover, the present volume includes detailed lists of medical illnesses and drugs that sometimes cause depression and anxiety, and a brief psychosocial interview and a guide to assess current psychosocial functioning.

THE 5 MINUTE PSYCHIATRIC SCREENING INTERVIEW

The 5 minute psychiatric screening interview is a mental health review of systems covering most of the major axis I disorders. The screening questions are linked to specific diagnostic categories (printed in bold above the questions). In parentheses are the page numbers in the guide for the complete set of questions for that disorder. This review of systems should be prefaced by an introduction of the type given below.

****

One of the most important parts of a person's well being is their emotional health. Stress and nerves have a big influence on many of my patients physical problems. I want to take a few minutes now to understand how you deal with life stress and whether anything is bothering you emotionally. I know that it's sometimes difficult to talk about these things. In fact, during the past few years doctors have learned that a large number of their patients are bothered by clinical anxiety or depression that never gets properly diagnosed or treated.

Major Depression/Dysthymia (pages 34-39)

> Let me begin by asking about your mood. How would you describe your mood?
> Have you been feeling sad, blue, down, or depressed?
> Have you lost interest in, or do you get less pleasure from, the things you used to enjoy?

Mania/Hypomania (pages 30-33)

> Have there been times lasting at least a few days when you felt the opposite of depressed, that is when you were very cheerful or high and this felt different than your normal self?
> > **IF NO:** What about a period lasting at least a couple of days when you were unusually irritable, and quick to argue or fight?

Generalized Anxiety Disorder (pages 48-49)

> What about feeling nervous or tense?
> Are you generally a nervous person?
> Are you a worrier?

Panic Disorder (pages 40-41)

Have you ever had an anxiety or panic attack in which you had a sudden, unexpected, rush of very intense fear or anxiety?

Social Phobia (pages 44-45)

Some people have very strong fears of being judged or evaluated by others. For example, a fear of eating or writing in front of others, public speaking, saying something foolish in a group of people, etc. Do you worry that you might do or say something that would embarass you in front of others?

Specific Phobia (pages 46-47)

Some people have very strong fears or phobias of certain situations such as heights, flying, bugs, snakes, etc. Do you have any very strong fears or phobias?

Agoraphobia (pages 42-43)

What about fears of bridges, tunnels, going outside alone, being at home alone, or other places or situations?

Obsessions (pages 58-60)

Some people are frequently bothered by intrusive, silly, unpleasant, or horrible thoughts that seem unreasonable or do not make sense, but they keep repeating over and over. For example, repeated thoughts that you might hurt or kill someone you love, even though you didn't want to; that someone you love is hurt; that you will yell obscenities in public; that you are contaminated by germs or dirt; or that you just hit someone while driving. Has anything like this been a problem for you?

Body Dysmorphic Disorder (page 66)

Do you often think there is something wrong with the way you look?
Do you often think you look gross, disfigured, or ugly?

Compulsions (pages 59-60)

Some people are frequently bothered by having to do something over and over that they can't resist when they try. For example, they wash their hands repeatedly, check whether the door is locked or the stove is turned off, or count things excessively. Has this been a problem for you?

Trichotillomania (page 67)

Some people feel compelled to pull out their hair. Do you frequently pull out enough hair from your head, eyebrows, or other parts of your body that it is noticeable (to others)?

Alcohol Abuse/Dependence (pages 12-15)

Now I'm going to ask a few questions about your use of alcohol. What are your drinking habits like?
Was there ever a time in your life when you drank too much?
Has anyone in your family, friends, a doctor, or anyone else ever said that you were an excessive drinker?
Has alcohol ever caused problems for you?

Drug Abuse/Dependence (pages 16-21)

What about street drugs? Have you ever used street drugs?
Did you or anyone else ever think you used drugs too much?
Did you ever use sleeping pills, weight loss medicines, or painkillers?
   IF YES: Did you ever get hooked on them or take more than was prescribed?

Bulimia (pages 10-11)

Now let me ask a couple of questions about your eating habits. Have you ever gone on eating binges when you ate an abnormally large amount of food over a short period of time?
   IF YES: Did you feel you lost control of your eating?

Anorexia Nervosa (pages 8-9)

Has there ever been a time when people gave you a hard time about being too thin or losing too much weight?

Posttraumatic Stress Disorder (pages 50-53)

> Earlier, I asked a little bit about recent stressors. Considering your entire life, have you ever seen or experienced a traumatic event in which your life was actually in danger, or you thought your life was in danger?
> **IF YES:** What happened?

Psychosis (pages 26-29)

> And finally, does your mind ever play tricks on you so that you hear things that other people don't hear, or see things they don't see?
> Do you ever feel like someone's spying on you or plotting to hurt you?
> Do you have any ideas that you don't like to talk about because you're afraid other people will think you're crazy?

****

To reiterate, the preceding are screening questions for the disorders described in the rest of this book. Positive responses need to be clarified and followed up with questions assessing the full set of diagnostic criteria.

Screening questions are not included for hypochondriasis and somatization disorder because they should not be asked in a separate mental health review of systems, but instead should be incorporated into the medical history (See pages 64-65 for hypochondriasis, and 61-63 for somatization disorder).

ANOREXIA NERVOSA

> Inclusion: A-D (In men: A-C)
> Exclusion: None

(A) Refusal to maintain body weight at or above a minimally normal weight for age and height (e.g., weight loss leading to maintenance of body weight less than 85% of that expected; or failure to make expected weight gain during period of growth, leading to body weight less than 85% of that expected).

Has there ever been a time when people gave you a hard time about being too thin or losing too much weight?
Have you ever weighed much less than people thought you should weigh?

IF YES TO EITHER QUESTION:
When did this occur?
Is this still true?
What was the lowest you weighed?
How tall were you?
What do you weigh now?

(B) Intense fear of gaining weight or becoming fat, even though underweight.

During the time you weighed less than others thought you should weigh, were you very afraid of gaining weight or becoming fat?

(C) Disturbance in the way in which one's body weight or shape is experienced; undue influence of body weight or shape on self-evaluation, or denial of the seriousness of the current low body weight.

During that time, how did you think your body looked?
Did other people say you were thin, but you thought you <u>looked</u> fat or overweight?
Did your body <u>feel</u> fat?
   IF YES: Any particular part?

Did your weight or the shape of your body have a big effect on your opinion of yourself? **IF YES:** Tell me about that.

How much did you think about the health risks of weighing (LOWEST WEIGHT)?

(D)	In postmenarcheal females, amenorrhea, i.e., the absence of at least three consecutive menstrual cycles. (A woman is considered to have amenorrhea if her periods occur only following hormone, e.g., estrogen, administration).

When you were very thin or losing weight did you start missing some of your menstrual periods?
    IF YES: How often?
              Did you ever miss 3 in a row?

BULIMIA NERVOSA

> Inclusion: A-D
> Exclusion: E

(A) Recurrent episodes of binge eating as characterized by both: 1) eating, in a discrete period of time (e.g., within any two hour period), an amount of food that is definitely larger than most people would eat during a similar period of time and under similar circumstances, and 2) a sense of lack of control over eating during the episode (e.g., a feeling that one cannot stop eating or control what or how much one is eating).

---

1) Have you ever gone on eating binges when you ate abnormally large amounts of food over a short period of time?
   IF YES: How much would you eat during a binge?

2) During a binge did you feel you lost control of your eating?

(B) Recurrent inappropriate compensatory behavior in order to prevent weight gain, such as self-induced vomiting; misuse of laxatives, diuretics, enemas, or other medications; fasting; or excessive exercise.

To prevent gaining weight from the binge, would you sometimes...
   ...force yourself to vomit?
   ...go on strict diets or fast afterwards?
   ...use laxatives or water pills?
   ...give yourself an enema?
   ...exercise vigorously?
   IF YES TO ANY: Describe what that was like.

(C) The binge eating and inappropriate compensatory behaviors both occur, on average, at least twice a week for three months.

How often did you binge?

Was there ever a time lasting at least 3 months when you would binge at least twice a week?

How often did you [COMPENSATORY BEHAVIOR]?
Did you ever do this at least twice a week for 3 or more months?

(D)	**Self-evaluation is unduly influenced by body shape and weight.**

Did your weight or the shape of your body have a big effect on your opinion of yourself?
  IF YES: Tell me about that.

(E)	<u>Exclude</u> **the diagnosis if the symptoms occur exclusively during episodes of anorexia nervosa.**

IF ANOREXIC: Did you also binge and [COMPENSATORY BEHAVIOR] when you weren't underweight like you were when you were [AGE]?

ALCOHOL ABUSE/DEPENDENCE

> Alcohol Dependence: at least 3 from B
> Alcohol Abuse: at least 1 from A, not dependent

Screening Questions

Now I'm going to ask you some questions about your use of alcohol.
What are your drinking habits like?
Was there ever a time in your life when you drank too much?
 IF YES: How old were you?
Has anyone in your family ever said that you were an excessive drinker?
Have friends, a doctor, or anyone else ever said that you drink too much?
Has alcohol ever caused problems for you?
 IF YES: What kind of problems?
     How old were you when you had these problems?

**If all of the above questions are ANSWERED NO,
the diagnosis of alcohol abuse/dependence is unlikely.**

The following questions deal with the time you were drinking the most, and having the most problems with your drinking.

A. **Alcohol Abuse:** A maladaptive pattern of alcohol use leading to clinically significant impairment or distress, as manifested by one or more of the following occurring within a twelve month period:

(A1) Recurrent alcohol use resulting in a failure to fulfill major role obligations at work, school, or home (e.g., repeated absences or poor work performance related to alcohol use; alcohol related absences, suspensions, or expulsions from school; neglect of children or household).

Because of drinking, how often did you...

....miss work (or school)?
....have trouble at work (or school)?
....get fired (or suspended or expelled from school)?
....not take care of children?
....not cook, clean the house, or go grocery shopping?

Alcohol Abuse/Dependence

(A2) Recurrent alcohol use in situations in which it is physically hazardous (e.g., driving an automobile or operating a machine when impaired by alcohol use).

Did you drive while intoxicated? **IF YES:** How often?

Did you ever drink and then do something that was potentially physically dangerous (e.g., operate machinery)?

(A3) Recurrent alcohol-related legal problems (e.g. arrest for disorderly conduct).

Were you ever arrested for driving under the influence, or disorderly conduct? **IF YES:** How many times?

(A4) Continued alcohol use despite having persistent or recurrent social or interpersonal problems caused or exacerbated by the effects of the alcohol (e.g., arguments with spouse about consequences of intoxication, physical fights).

Because of your drinking did you...
...frequently have problems or arguments with friends or family?
...spend less time with family or friends?
...get separated or divorced?
...get into physical fights?
...get violent?
IF YES TO ANY: Did you still drink despite these problems?

B. **Alcohol Dependence:** A maladaptive pattern of alcohol use, leading to clinically significant impairment or distress, as manifested by three or more of the following occurring at any time in the same twelve month period:

(B1) Tolerance, as defined by either: 1) need for markedly increased amounts of alcohol to achieve intoxication or desired effect, or 2) markedly diminished effect with continued use of the same amount of alcohol.

1) Over time did you drink a lot more to get high or get the same effect as before? **IF YES:** How much more?

2) Did you develop a tolerance to alcohol so that the same amount as previously did not have the same effect?

(B2) Withdrawal, as manifested by either: 1) within several hours to a few days after cessation or reduction of heavy and prolonged alcohol use, person experienced at least two characteristic symptoms of withdrawal, or 2) alcohol (or related substance) often taken to relieve or avoid withdrawal symptoms.

1) Did any of the following occur when you quit or cut down your drinking:
   1) Heart racing or sweating
   2) The shakes
   3) Sleep problems
   4) Nausea or vomiting
   5) Seeing, hearing, or feeling things that weren't really there (hallucinations)
   6) Feeling fidgety, restless, or agitated
   7) Anxiety or nervousness
   8) Seizures
   IF YES TO ANY: How soon after you quit or cut down did the [SYMPTOM] begin?

2) Did you often drink or take anything else to stop withdrawal symptoms, or to prevent them from coming on? (Did you drink in the morning to stop withdrawal symptoms from coming on?)

(B3) Alcohol is often taken in larger amounts or over a longer period than the person intended.

When you drank, did you often drink more than you had planned?

When you drank, did you often drink for more time than you had planned?

(B4) Persistent desire or unsuccessful efforts to cut down or control alcohol use.

Did you frequently think about cutting down or stopping drinking?
   IF YES: How much did you think about that?
   For how long did you think about that? (Week? Months?)

At times, did you try to cut down or stop but couldn't?
   IF NO: For example, some people try to control their drinking by promising not to begin before a certain time or not to drink alone. Did you ever do things like that?
   IF YES: How often would you try to cut back or stop completely?

Alcohol Abuse/Dependence 15

(B5) **A great deal of time is spent in activities necessary to get alcohol (e.g., driving long distances), drinking alcohol, or recovering from its effects.**

Did you spend a lot of time doing things and planning ways to get alcohol? **IF YES:** Was this the number one thing on your mind?

How much time did you spend drinking?

How often were you intoxicated?

Did you spend a lot of time recovering from hangovers?

(B6) **Important social, occupational, or recreational activities given up or reduced because of alcohol use.**

Did you spend so much of your time drinking that you...
 ...missed a lot of time from work?
 ...spent less time with family or friends?
 ...gave up some hobbies or other interests?
IF YES: Tell me about that.

(B7) **Continued alcohol use despite knowledge of having had a persistent or recurrent physical or psychological problem that was likely to have been caused or exacerbated by the alcohol (e.g., continued drinking despite recognition that an ulcer was made worse by the alcohol consumption).**

Did drinking cause physical problems?
 IF YES: Like what?
  Did you continue to drink despite these problems?

Did drinking cause anxiety or depression?
 IF YES: Did you still drink anyway?

Did drinking cause any other type of psychological problem?
 IF YES: Like what?
  Did you continue to drink despite these problems?

DRUG ABUSE/DEPENDENCE

> Drug Dependence: at least 3 from B
> Drug Abuse: at least 1 from A, not dependent

Screening Questions

Street Drugs

Have you ever used any street drugs?
 IF YES: What? How frequently?

> ***IF USED LESS THAN 10 TIMES IN LIFE, SKIP TO SCREENING QUESTIONS REGARDING PRESCRIBED MEDICINES***
>
> Did you ever think that you used drugs too much?
> **IF YES:** How old were you?
> Has anyone in your family ever said that you've used drugs too much?
> Have friends, a doctor, or anyone else ever said that you used drugs too much?
> Have drugs ever caused problems for you?
> **IF YES:** What kinds of problems?
>   How old were you when you had these problems?

Prescribed Medication

Have you ever used sleeping pills, tranquilizers, weight loss medicines, or painkillers?
 IF YES: How long did you take [DRUG]?
   Did you get hooked or addicted to it?
   Did you ever take much more than was prescribed?

If all of the above questions are ANSWERED NO, the diagnosis of drug abuse/dependence is unlikely.

The following questions deal with the time you were using drugs the most, and having the most problems with your drug use.

Drug Abuse/Dependence 17

A. <u>Drug Abuse</u>: **A maladaptive pattern of drug use leading to clinically significant impairment or distress, as manifested by one or more of the following occurring within a twelve month period:**

(A1) Recurrent drug use resulting in a failure to fulfill major role obligations at work, school, or home (e.g., repeated absences or poor work performance related to drug use; drug related absences, suspensions, or expulsions from school; neglect of children or household).

Because of your [DRUG] use, how often did you...
....miss work (or school)?
....have trouble at work (or school)?
....get fired (or suspended or expelled from school)?
....not take care of children?
....not cook, clean the house, or go grocery shopping?

(A2) Recurrent drug use in situations in which it is physically hazardous (e.g., driving an automobile or operating a machine when impaired by drug use).

Did you frequently drive while high on drugs? **IF YES:** How often?

Did you ever use drugs and then do something that was potentially physically dangerous (e.g., operate machinery)?

(A3) Recurrent drug-related legal problems.

Were you ever arrested or busted for using or selling drugs?
   IF YES: How many times?

(A4) Continued drug use despite having persistent or recurrent social or interpersonal problems caused or exacerbated by the effects of the drug use (e.g., arguments with spouse about consequences of drug use, physical fights).

Because of your [DRUG] use did you...
...frequently have problems or arguments with friends or family?
...spend less time with family or friends?
...get separated or divorced?
...get into physical fights?
   IF YES TO ANY: Did you still use drugs despite these problems?

18 *Drug Abuse/Dependence*

B. **Drug Dependence:** A maladaptive pattern of drug use, leading to clinically significant impairment or distress, as manifested by three or more of the following, occurring at any time in the same twelve month period:

(B1) **Tolerance**, as defined by <u>either</u>: 1) a need for markedly increased amount of the drug to achieve intoxication or desired effect, or 2) markedly diminished effect with continued use of the same amount of the drug.

---

1) Over time did you use a lot more to get high or get the same effect as before? **IF YES:** How much more?

2) Did you develop a tolerance to [DRUG] so that the same amount as previously did not have the same effect?

****
NOTE: Criterion B2 refers to withdrawal from substances. Withdrawal symptoms vary according to the class of substance. Below, questions are separately listed to determine withdrawal from three classes of substances--stimulants, opioids, and sedatives.
****

(B2) <u>**Amphetamine/stimulant or cocaine withdrawal**</u>, as manifested by <u>either</u>: 1) within a few hours to a several days after cessation or reduction of prolonged and heavy stimulant or cocaine use, person experienced dysphoric mood (item 1), and at least two other characteristic symptoms of withdrawal, or 2) substance (or related substance) often taken to relieve or avoid withdrawal symptoms.

---

1) Did any of the following occur when you quit or cut down on your use of [SUBSTANCE]:
   1) Depressed, irritable, or anxious mood
   2) Fatigue
   3) Vivid, unpleasant dreams
   4) Increased or decreased sleep
   5) Increased appetite
   6) Feeling very slowed down like you were stuck in mud, or the reverse, feeling restless and agitated
      IF YES TO ANY: How soon after you quit or cut down did the [SYMPTOM] begin?
2) Did you often use drugs to stop withdrawal symptoms or to prevent them from coming on?

Drug Abuse/Dependence 19

(B2) <u>Opioid withdrawal</u>, as manifested by <u>either</u>: 1) within minutes to a few days after cessation or reduction of prolonged and heavy opioid use, or administration of an opioid antagonist, person experienced at least three characteristic symptoms of withdrawal, or 2) substance often taken to relieve or avoid withdrawal symptoms.

---

1) Did any of the following occur when you quit or cut down on your use of [SUBSTANCE]:
   1) Depressed or irritable mood
   2) Nausea or vomiting
   3) Muscle aches
   4) Tearing or runny nose
   5) Dilated pupils, goose bumps, or sweating
   6) Diarrhea
   7) Yawning
   8) Fever
   9) Decreased sleep
      IF YES TO ANY: How soon after you quit or cut down did the [SYMPTOM] begin?
2) Did you often use drugs to stop withdrawal symptoms or to prevent them from coming on?

(B2) <u>Sedative, hypnotic, or anxiolytic withdrawal</u>, as manifested by <u>either</u>: 1) within several hours to a few days after cessation or reduction of prolonged and heavy substance use, person experienced at least two characteristic symptoms of withdrawal, or 2) substance often taken to relieve or avoid withdrawal symptoms.

---

1) Did any of the following occur when you quit or cut down on your use of [SUBSTANCE]:
   1) Heart racing or sweating
   2) The shakes
   3) Sleep problems
   4) Nausea or vomiting
   5) Seeing, hearing, or feeling things that weren't really there (hallucinations)
   6) Feeling fidgety, restless, or agitated
   7) Anxiety or nervousness
   8) Seizures
      IF YES TO ANY: How soon after you quit or cut down did the [SYMPTOM] begin?
2) Did you often use drugs, or drink alcohol, to stop withdrawal symptoms or to prevent them from coming on?

Drug Abuse/Dependence

(B3) The drug is often taken in larger amounts or over a longer period than the person intended.

When you used [DRUG], did you often use more than you had planned?

When you used [DRUG], did you often use it for a longer period of time than you had planned?

(B4) Persistent desire or unsuccessful efforts to cut down or control drug use.

Did you frequently think about cutting down or stopping your use of [DRUG]? **IF YES:** How much did you think about that?

At times, did you try to cut down or stop but couldn't?
  IF NO: For example, some people try to control their drug use by promising not to begin before a certain time or not to use drugs alone. Did you ever do things like that?
  IF YES: How often would you try to cut back or stop completely?

(B5) A great deal of time is spent in activities necessary to get drugs (e.g., visiting multiple doctors, driving long distances), using drugs, or recovering from its effects.

Did you spend a lot of time doing things and planning ways to get drugs? **IF YES:** Was this the number one thing on your mind?

How much time did you spend using [DRUG]?

How often were you high?

Did you spend a lot of time recovering from using [DRUG]?

(B6) Important social, occupational, or recreational activities given up or reduced because of drug use.

Did you spend so much of your time getting high that you...
  ...missed a lot of time from work?
  ...spent less time with family or friends?
  ...gave up some hobbies or other interests?
IF YES: Tell me about that.

(B7) Continued drug use despite knowledge of having had a persistent or recurrent physical or psychological problem that was likely to have been caused or exacerbated by the drugs (e.g., continued cocaine use despite recognition of cocaine-induced depression).

Did using [DRUG] cause physical problems?
    IF YES: Like what?
              Did you continue to use [DRUG] despite these problems?

Did using [DRUG] cause anxiety or depression?
    IF YES: Did you still use [DRUG] anyway?

Did using [DRUG] cause any other type of psychological problem?
    IF YES: Like what?
              Did you continue to use [DRUG] despite these problems?

SCHIZOPHRENIA AND OTHER PSYCHOTIC DISORDERS

Primary care physicians do not frequently treat acutely and overtly psychotic patients. However, in its earliest stages, psychosis may not be so severe, and early identification may prevent the devastating psychosocial consequences of florid psychosis. Consequently, I have included this section on the psychotic disorders.

The diagnostic criteria for schizophrenia are complex and involve 1) inquiry for delusions and hallucinations, 2) inquiry for manic and depressive syndromes and if these have been present, then determining whether they are brief relative to the duration of illness, 3) inquiry for the duration of the active psychotic symptom phase, as well as the residual and prodromal illness phases, 4) inquiry to determine deterioration in level of functioning, and 5) observation of affective, behavioral, and cognitive signs of the illness.

The user of this guide should refer to the DSM-IV manual to fully appreciate the differences between schizophrenia, delusional disorder, schizophreniform disorder, brief psychotic disorder and schizoaffective disorder. The common thread to these disorders is the presence of psychosis. Unlike the other sections of this guide, the questions do not follow the DSM-IV diagnostic algorithms. Instead, I briefly summarize the salient features of these disorders, and then highlight differential diagnosis considerations for five pairs of disorders. The questions for detecting delusions and hallucinations are listed on pages 26-29.

<u>Schizophrenia</u> is generally a chronic illness beginning before the age of 25 in which the individual does not return to his or her premorbid level of functioning. Prominent hallucinations or bizarre delusions are usually present. The person must be ill at least six months, though they need not be actively psychotic all of the time. Three phases of the illness are defined. The prodrome phase refers to a deterioration in function prior to the onset of the active psychotic phase. The active phase symptoms (delusions, hallucinations, disorganized speech, grossly disorganized behavior, or negative symptoms such as flat affect) must be present for at least one month. The residual phase follows the active phase. The features of the residual and prodromal phases include functional impairment, and abnormalities in affect, cognition, and communication. If a manic or depressive syndrome occurs, its duration is brief relative to the duration of the active phase of schizophrenia. (DSM-IV does not

indicate how short the mood syndrome must be to be considered "brief". I will not diagnose schizophrenia if a full mood syndrome has been present during more than 10-20% of the active phase of the illness.)

The DSM-IV definition of schizophrenia has 5 criteria. Criterion A, or the active phase of illness, requires the presence of <u>two</u> of the following features for at least one month: delusions, hallucinations, disorganized speech, grossly disorganized or catatonic behavior, and negative symptoms. Of note, only one of these features is required if the delusions are bizarre, or if there are auditory hallucinations consisting of either a voice keeping up a running commentary on the person's behavior or thoughts, or two or more voices conversing with each other. Criterion B refers to social or occupational impairment, and Criterion C refers to the six month duration of disturbance. Criteria D and E exclude the diagnosis if there is significant mood disorder pathology, or if the disturbance is due to the effects of street drugs, medication, or medical illness.

<u>Delusional Disorder</u> is also usually a chronic illness. The delusions last at least a month and are <u>not</u> bizarre but instead involve situations that can occur in real life such as infidelity, being followed, illness, etc. Hallucinations, if present, are not prominent. Functional impairment is directly linked to the delusional system. Often functioning is not markedly and pervasively impaired. If a manic or depressive syndrome occurs, its duration is brief relative to the duration of the delusions.

<u>Brief Psychotic Disorder</u> requires the presence of <u>one</u> of the following for at least one day but less than a month: delusions, hallucinations, disorganized speech, or grossly disorganized or catatonic behavior. The individual returns to his or her normal self.

<u>Schizophreniform Disorder</u> lasts at least one month, but less than six months, is characterized by delusions, prominent hallucinations, or the other active phase features of schizophrenia, and a manic or depressive syndrome, if present, must be brief relative to the duration of the psychotic symptoms. Thus, the criteria are similar to those of schizophrenia except the illness duration is less than six months, and there is no social or occupational impairment requirement.

<u>Schizoaffective Disorder</u> is diagnosed when the patient has the characteristic features of the active phase of schizophrenia, but the duration of the manic or depressive syndrome is <u>not</u> brief relative to the duration of the psychosis. However, for at least two weeks the individual has delusions or hallucinations but not prominent mood symptoms (and this excludes the diagnosis of a mood disorder).

DIFFERENTIATING PSYCHOTIC DISORDERS

1. **Schizophrenia vs. Delusional Disorder:** In delusional disorder, the content of the delusions involve events that may actually occur to some people in real life (e.g., being followed by the FBI, having cancer, becoming a famous entertainer or author, being poisoned, etc.). Bizarre delusions such as thought broadcasting and delusions of control, and prominent hallucinations, only occur in schizophrenia. Hallucinations can occur in individuals with delusional disorder; however, they are limited to a few brief periods. Similarly, disorganized speech, grossly disorganized or catatonic behavior, and negative symptoms are usually absent in delusional disorder (or if present, they are present for less than a few hours). Thus, criterion A of schizophrenia is <u>not</u> present. Nonbizarre delusions can occur in schizophrenia; however, they are not the only psychotic symptom. The individual with schizophrenia additionally experiences either bizarre delusions, prominent hallucinations, or markedly disturbed affect, thought processes, or behavior.

2. **Schizophrenia vs. Schizoaffective Disorder:** The psychotic symptoms are the same. In schizoaffective disorder a manic or depressive episode <u>must be present</u>, and the duration of the mood syndrome is <u>not brief</u> relative to the duration of the psychosis. (As noted above, DSM-IV does not define "brief duration.") However, to be diagnosed with schizoaffective disorder there must be at least two weeks in which the delusions or hallucinations are present but prominent mood symptoms are not.

3. **Schizoaffective Disorder vs. Mood Disorder with Psychotic Features:** In a psychotic mood disorder, there are no periods (or only very brief ones) characterized by psychosis but without prominent mood symptoms. You cannot rely on the content and type of psychotic symptoms, or the number and severity of mood symptoms, to distinguish these two disorders. Rather, the distinguishing factor is whether or not the psychotic and mood symptoms overlap in time.

4. **Schizophrenia vs. Schizophreniform Disorder:** The symptom inclusion criteria are the same. The primary difference is that schizophrenia lasts for more than six months (including the prodromal, active, and residual phases), whereas in schizophreniform disorder the pathology (i.e., all three phases) has lasted less than six months.

5. **Schizophreniform Disorder vs. Brief Psychotic Disorder:** Both refer to psychotic disorders of brief duration. The psychotic symptom inclusion criteria are similar, but not identical. The psychosis inclusion criteria are broader for brief psychotic disorder (any one of: delusions, hallucinations, disorganized speech, grossly disorganized behavior or speech <u>versus</u> criterion A of schizophrenia which requires at least two of five features (unless the delusions or hallucinations are of a special nature, in which case only one feature is required)). Schizophreniform disorder lasts at least a month, whereas brief psychotic disorder lasts less than a month.

ASSESSING DELUSIONS AND HALLUCINATIONS

DELUSION OF REFERENCE

When watching TV, listening to the radio, or reading the paper do you notice that they are referring to you, or that there are special messages intended specifically for you?
IF YES: What have you noticed?

Does it seem like strangers on the street are taking special notice of you or talking about you?
IF YES: Is it a feeling you have, or are you pretty sure that they are talking about/referring to you?
IF PRETTY SURE: How do you know?

Do things seem especially arranged for you?
IF YES: In what way?

DELUSION OF PERSECUTION

Is anybody against you, following you, giving you a hard time, or trying to hurt you?
IF YES: Tell me about that.

Do you feel like there's a plot to hurt you?
IF YES: Who's involved?
Why would they want to hurt you?

THOUGHT BROADCASTING

Do you ever think of something so strongly that people could hear your thoughts?
IF YES: So, people can hear what you are thinking even when you're not talking?
How do you know?

DELUSION OF MIND READING

Are people able to read your mind and know what you're thinking?
IF YES: How can they do this?
Can anyone do it, or just some people? Who?
Do they literally read your thoughts, or do they read your facial expression to know what you're thinking?

THOUGHT WITHDRAWAL

Are your thoughts ever taken out of your head?
IF DOESN'T UNDERSTAND QUESTION:
Does someone or some force reach into your head and steal or remove your thoughts?

IF YES TO EITHER QUESTION:
Tell me about it.

THOUGHT INSERTION

Are there ever thoughts in your head that have been put in there from the outside?
IF YES: Tell me about it.
(I'm not referring to talking to someone who makes a suggestion or gives you advice. Instead I'm referring to thoughts getting inserted into your head from the outside. Does this ever happen?)

DELUSION OF GUILT

(Also see major depression section, page 36)
Do you think you've done something terrible and deserve to be punished?
IF YES: I know it will be hard to talk about, but what do you feel so guilty about?

Do you blame yourself for bad things going on in the world like wars, crime, starvation, etc.?

DELUSION OF GRANDIOSITY

(See Mania section, page 31)

DELUSION OF CONTROL

Do you ever get the feeling that you're being controlled by some force or power from the outside?
IF YES: What's that like?
   At times, does it seem like you're not in control of your body, almost like you're a puppet and something from the outside pulls the strings?
   IF YES: So, at times your body does certain things without your willing it?
      IF YES: If I asked you to raise your hand or stand up now would you be able to do it?
         IF NO: Why is that?
         IF YES: So, you're in control of your actions? Are you always in control?

SOMATIC DELUSION

Are you concerned that you have a serious physical illness that a doctor hasn't found, or that something is wrong with your body?
IF YES: What do you think is wrong?
   Why do you think that?
   Are you sure?

****
HALLUCINATIONS
****

VISUAL HALLUCINATIONS

Have you seen visions or other things that other people didn't see?
IF YES: What did you see?
   What time of the day did this occur?
   How long ago did it start?
   Do you see it every day?
   How often do you see it?

AUDITORY HALLUCINATIONS

Have you heard noises, or sounds, or voices that other people didn't hear?
- **IF YES:** What did you hear?
    - Do the voices seem to come from inside or outside your head? **IF INSIDE:** But you hear it with your ears?
    - How many voices do you hear?
    - Are they male or female? Do you recognize them?
    - Do you ever hear two or more voices talking to each other?
    - Do the voices ever talk about what you're doing or thinking?
        - **IF YES:** Do they ever keep up a running commentary on what you're doing or thinking just like a sports announcer describes a ballgame?
    - How long ago did the voices start?
    - Do you hear them every day?
    - How often during the day do you hear them?
    - Do they influence your behavior?
    - Do they tell you to do things?

TACTILE HALLUCINATIONS

Do you ever notice strange sensations in your body or on your skin?

Do you ever feel something creeping or crawling on your body, or something push or punch you but no one is there?
- **IF YES:** Like what?
    - When did it happen the first time?
    - How often has it happened?

OLFACTORY AND GUSTATORY HALLUCINATIONS

What about smells that other people don't notice, or strange tastes in your mouth?
- **IF YES:** Like what?
    - When did it happen the first time?
    - How often has it happened?
    - Are they associated with any other physical symptoms like an upset stomach, numbness, tingling, or brief memory loss?
        - **IF YES:** Tell me about that.

MANIA/HYPOMANIA

> Inclusion:* A, at least 3 or 4 from B, C
> Exclusion: D, E

*Diagnostic Note: 1) In diagnosing mania and hypomania at least 3 items are required from B if the predominant mood is euphoric, at least 4 items are required if the predominant mood is irritable.

(A) **MANIA:** A distinct period of abnormally and persistently elevated, expansive, or irritable mood, lasting at least one week (or any duration if hospitalization is necessary).

(A) **HYPOMANIA:** A distinct period of persistently elevated, expansive, or irritable mood, lasting throughout at least four days, that is clearly different from the usual nondepressed mood.

Have there been times lasting at least a few days when you felt the opposite of depressed, that is when you were very cheerful or high and this felt different than your normal self?
IF YES OR UNCLEAR:
Did you feel hyper, or like you were high on drugs, even though you hadn't taken anything?
Did anything cause your good mood?
How long did it last?
So, was this more than just feeling good?
When did this occur?
How many periods like this have you had?
IF NO: What about a period lasting at least a few days when you were unusually irritable, and quick to argue or fight?
IF YES: Describe what that was like.
Were you using drugs or alcohol?
Did you get into many arguments or fights?
How long did this period last?
Was there a reason you felt that way?
When did it occur?
How many periods like this have you had?

Now I'm going to ask about some other things that you might have been thinking or feeling when you were feeling [HIGH, HYPER, EUPHORIC, IRRITABLE, etc.]...

B. During the period of mood disturbance, at least three of the following have persisted (four if the mood is only irritable) and have been present to a significant degree:

(B1) Inflated self-esteem or grandiosity.

What was your self-esteem like during this time?

Did you feel more self-confident than usual?

Did you think you had special talents, abilities, or powers?
   IF YES: Like what?

When some people feel [HIGH, EUPHORIC, etc.] they may think they're going to become famous or do great things. Did you have any thoughts like that? IF YES: Like what?

(B2) Decreased need for sleep (e.g., feels rested after only three hours of sleep).

During this time, how did you sleep?

Did you need less sleep than usual in order to feel rested?

(B3) More talkative than usual or pressure to keep talking.

Were you more talkative than usual?

Did you talk on and on so that people couldn't shut you up or interrupt?

Did you feel a pressure to talk constantly?

Did you talk faster than normal?
   IF YES: Did you talk so fast that people couldn't understand you?

(B4) Flight of ideas or subjective experience that thoughts are racing.

During this time, did it feel like your thoughts were going very fast and racing through your mind?

Mania/Hypomania

(B5) Distractibility (i.e., attention too easily drawn to unimportant or irrelevant external stimuli).

Were you easily distracted so that any little thing could get you off track? **IF YES:** What was that like?

(B6) Increase in goal-directed activity (either socially, at work or school, or sexually) or psychomotor agitation.

Were you more active than usual? For example, did you do more chores around the house?

Were you so energetic that instead of sleeping you did household chores or work throughout the night?

Did you start new projects or take on added responsibilities?

Did you work more?

Did you call friends more?

Were you sexually more active than usual?

Did you feel physically restless so that it was hard to sit still and you were always moving or pacing back and forth?
 IF YES TO ANY OF ABOVE: Tell me what you did.

(B7) Excessive involvement in pleasurable activities that have a high potential for painful consequences (e.g., engaging in unrestrained buying sprees, sexual indiscretions, or foolish business investments).

Did you do anything that could have caused problems for you or your family? For example, when some people feel [MANIC MOOD] they go on spending sprees, write bad checks, invest money foolishly, or do things sexually that are unusual for them. Did you do anything like that? **IF YES:** Like what?

(C) <u>MANIA:</u> The mood disturbance is sufficiently severe to cause marked impairment in occupational functioning or in usual social activities or relationships with others, or to necessitate hospitalization to prevent harm to self or others, or there are psychotic features.

Mania/Hypomania

(C) **HYPOMANIA:** The episode is associated with an unequivocal change in functioning that is uncharacteristic of the person when not symptomatic, and the disturbance in mood and change in functioning is observable by others.

Did anyone notice that there was something different about you?
 IF YES: What did they say?
 IF NO: Did anyone notice [MANIA SYMPTOMS NOTED ABOVE]?

What effect did this episode have on your life at the time it was going on?

Did it cause major problems in your job (school)?....marriage? ....relationships with friends or family?....social life?
 IF YES TO ANY ITEM: What happened?

Did anyone notice that you weren't functioning the way you normally do?
 IF YES: What did they say?

Did you get treatment?
 IF YES: Were you hospitalized?

(D) <u>Exclude</u> the diagnosis if during the course of the illness the patient had delusions or hallucinations for at least two weeks in the absence of prominent mood symptoms. In such cases the diagnosis is schizophrenia, schizoaffective disorder, delusional disorder, schizophreniform disorder, or psychotic disorder NOS.

(See pages 26-29 for psychosis questions.)
IF PSYCHOTIC:
 Was there a time when you [PSYCHOTIC SYMPTOM] but did not feel [MANIC MOOD] and have problems with [MANIC SYMPTOMS]?
  IF YES: How long did you have [PSYCHOTIC SYMPTOMS] only?
  When did the [MANIC MOOD AND SYMPTOMS] begin in relation to this?

(E) <u>Exclude</u> the diagnosis if the symptoms are due to physical illness (e.g., hyperthyroidism), or street drugs (amphetamines, cocaine).

MAJOR DEPRESSION

> Inclusion: A1 or A2, at least 5 from A, B
> Exclusion: C-E

NOTE: For each symptom you must inquire about duration (For how long have you...) and persistence (Do you feel like that nearly every day?).

NOTE: Do not include symptoms that are clearly due to a physical illness, or mood-incongruent delusions or hallucinations.

A. At least five of the following symptoms have been present during the same two week period and represent a change from previous functioning; at least one symptom is either 1) depressed mood or 2) loss of interest or pleasure.

(A1) Depressed mood most of the day, nearly every day, as indicated by either subjective report (e.g., feels sad or empty) or observation made by others (e.g., appears tearful).

How is your mood?
Have you been feeling sad, blue, down, or depressed?
  IF YES: For how long have you been feeling [DEPRESSED, DOWN, etc]?
  Do you feel that way nearly every day?
  How much of the day does it last?
  How bad is the feeling?

(A2) Markedly diminished interest or pleasure in all, or almost all, activities most of the day, nearly every day.

Have you lost interest in or do you get less pleasure from the things you used to enjoy?
  IF YES: What do you normally enjoy doing? (Television? Reading? Sports? Shopping? Socializing? Eating? Hobbies? Sex?)
  What do you still enjoy?
  What have you lost interest in?
  For how long have you not enjoyed these things like you used to?
  Is it like that nearly every day?

(A3) Significant weight loss when not dieting or weight gain (e.g., more than 5% of body weight in a month), or decrease or increase in appetite nearly every day.

Has there been any change in your appetite?
IF INCREASED OR DECREASED:
   How much more/less have you been eating?
   Is it like that nearly every day?
   For how long has your appetite been increased/decreased?

Have you gained/lost any weight? **IF YES:** How much? Since when?

(A4) Insomnia or hypersomnia nearly every day.

How have you been sleeping?
How many hours per night have you been sleeping?
How does this compare to normal?
IF INCREASED OR DECREASED:
   Is it a problem nearly every day?
   For how long have you had sleep problems?
      IF DECREASED: Do you have problems falling asleep, staying asleep, or waking up too early in the morning?

(A5) Psychomotor agitation or retardation nearly every day (observable by others, not merely subjective feelings of restlessness or being slowed down).

<u>Observation</u> of psychomotor agitation (fidgety while sitting; pacing; pulling on hair, skin, or clothing; handwringing; crossing and uncrossing legs frequently) and/or psychomotor retardation (slowed speech; long pauses before answering questions or between words; mute; slowed body movements) by interviewer or others.

Agitation: Have you been more fidgety and having problems sitting still?
   IF YES: Do you pace back and forth?
      Have others noticed your restlessness?

Retardation: Have you felt slowed down, like you were moving in slow motion or stuck in mud?
   IF YES: Have others noticed this?

(A6) Fatigue or loss of energy nearly every day.

How has your energy level been?
Have you been feeling tired or worn out?
> **IF YES:** Duration and persistence questions. (See top of pg. 34)

(A7) Feelings of worthlessness or excessive or inappropriate guilt nearly every day (not merely self-reproach or guilt about being sick).

How have you been feeling about yourself?
What's your self-esteem been like?
> **IF LOW:** What type of thoughts do you have about yourself?
> Do you feel like you're worthless or a failure?
> > **IF YES:** Tell me about it.

Have you been blaming yourself for things?
> **IF YES:** Like what?

Do you feel guilty?
> **IF YES:** About what?
> How hard is it to get your mind off of this?
> Do you think about things from the past and feel guilty about them?
> > **IF YES:** Like what?

IF EVIDENCE OF GUILT OR WORTHLESSNESS:
> How often do you actually think [PATIENT'S DESCRIPTION OF GUILT OR WORTHLESSNESS]? (Is this on your mind every day?)

(A8) Diminished ability to think or concentrate, or indecisiveness, nearly every day.

Have you been having problems thinking or concentrating?
> **IF YES:** What does this interfere with?
> Are you able to read? Watch TV? Follow a conversation?
> Duration and persistence questions.

Is it harder to make decisions than before?
> **IF YES:** What kind of decisions are harder to make?
> (What about everyday decisions?)
> Duration and persistence questions.

Major Depression

(A9)	**Recurrent thoughts of death (not just fear of dying), recurrent suicidal ideation without a specific plan, or a suicide attempt or a specific plan for committing suicide.**

> Sometimes when a person feels down or depressed they might think about dying. Have you been having any thoughts like that?
> **IF YES:** Tell me about it. Have you thought about taking your life?
> > **IF YES:** Did you think of a way to do it?
> > How close have you come to doing it?
> > **IF NO:** Do you wish you were dead?
> > When you go to sleep, do you often wish you would not wake up?

(B)	**The symptoms cause clinically significant distress or impairment in social, occupational, or other important areas of functioning.**

> What difficulties in your life has the depression caused?
> Does it bother you a lot that you feel this way?
> Has it caused problems in your job (school)?....marriage?
> ....relationships with friends or family?....social life?....doing household chores?

(C)	<u>Exclude</u> the diagnosis if the symptoms are due to physical illness (endocrine disorder), medication (antihypertensives), or street drugs (alcohol, cocaine withdrawal, PCP, steroids).

(D)	<u>Exclude</u> the diagnosis if the depression occurs within two months of the loss of a loved one (except if associated with marked functional impairment, morbid preoccupation with worthlessness, suicidal ideation, psychotic symptoms, or psychomotor retardation).

(E)	<u>Exclude</u> the diagnosis if during the course of the illness the patient had delusions or hallucinations for at least two weeks in the absence of prominent mood symptoms. In such cases the diagnosis is schizophrenia, schizoaffective disorder, delusional disorder, schizophreniform disorder, or psychotic disorder **NOS**.

> (See pages 26-29 for psychosis questions.)
> **IF PSYCHOTIC:**
> > Was there a time when you [PSYCHOTIC SX] but did not feel sad or depressed and have problems with [DEPRESSIVE SX]?
> > > **IF YES:** How long did you have [PSYCHOTIC SXS] only?
> > > When did the depression begin in relation to this?

DYSTHYMIC DISORDER

> Inclusion: A, at least 2 from B, C, H
> Exclusion: D-G

(A) Depressed mood for most of the day, for more days than not, as indicated by subjective account or observation of others for at least two years.

How is your mood?
Have you been feeling sad, blue, down, or depressed?
    IF YES: How often? (On more days than not?)
            For how long have you felt this way?
            (Has it been at least two years?)

Diagnostic Note: To diagnose dysthymia you must ensure that major depression has not been present during the past two years.

Recently, have you been more severely depressed than usual?
    IF NO: Was there a time in the past two years lasting at least two weeks when you felt more severely depressed than usual?
            IF YES TO EITHER: See pages 34-37 for major depression questions.

IF CURRENT MAJOR DEPRESSION:
For how long have you been feeling severely depressed with symptoms like [CURRENT DEPRESSIVE SYMPTOMS]? Before that, were you still bothered by a low level of depression?
    IF YES: Was that low level of depression present on most days?
            IF YES: So, even before this current episode of more severe depression, you were bothered by a milder depression on most days. Right?
                    For how long did you have the milder depression?

IF MAJOR DEPRESSION DURING PAST TWO YEARS:
Since you improved from your serious depression occurring last [DATE], have you still felt sad, blue, or depressed on most days?
    IF YES: Is that how you were before you got more severely depressed?
            IF YES: For how long before the serious depression were you bothered by the milder depression?

(B)	**Presence, while depressed, of at least two of the following:**

During this time (the time of the low level depression), do you often...
   1) ...have a poor appetite or overeat?
   2) ...have difficulty sleeping or with oversleeping?
   3) ...feel tired?
   4) ...feel down on yourself, or have low self-esteem?
   5) ...have problems concentrating or making decisions?
   6) ...feel hopeless or pessimistic about the future?

(C)	**During the two year period of the disturbance, never without the symptoms in A and B for more than two months at a time.**

During the [DYSTHYMIA TIME PERIOD] were you ever free of depression or sadness for a couple of months or more? Were you ever free of [SYMPTOMS IN B] for a couple of months or more?

(D)	<u>Exclude</u> the diagnosis if a major depression occurred during the first two years of the dysthymia.

When did the low level depression begin? See pages 34-37 for major depression questions, and determine if major depressive episode occurred during first two years of onset of dysthymia.

(E)	<u>Exclude</u> the diagnosis if the individual has a history of a manic or hypomanic episode.

(F)	<u>Exclude</u> diagnosis if the symptoms are superimposed on a chronic psychotic disorder such as schizophrenia or delusional disorder.

(G)	<u>Exclude</u> the diagnosis if the symptoms are due to the direct physiological effects of a substance (e.g., a drug of abuse, medication), or a general medical condition (e.g., hypothyroidism).

(H)	The symptoms cause clinically significant distress or impairment in social, occupational, or other important areas of functioning.

What difficulties in your life has the low level depression caused? Does it bother you a lot that you feel this way?
Has it caused problems in your job (school)?....marriage?
....relationships with friends or family?....social life?....doing household chores?

PANIC DISORDER

Inclusion: A
Exclusion: B, C

Diagnostic Note: Panic disorder can be diagnosed with or without agoraphobia. See pages 42-43 for agoraphobia questions.

(A) Recurrent unexpected panic attacks (see criteria for a panic attack on page 41), at least one of which has been followed by at least a month of one of the following: 1) persistent concern about having additional attacks, 2) worry about the implications of the attack or its consequences (e.g., losing control, having a heart attack, "going crazy"), or 3) a significant change in behavior related to the attacks.

An anxiety or panic attack is a sudden rush of intense fear, anxiety, or discomfort that comes on from out of the blue for no apparent reason, or in situations where you did not expect them to occur. Have you ever experienced this?
    IF YES: What was it like? (Ask about symptoms specified on page 41)
                How many attacks have you experienced?
                Do they ever awaken you from sleep?
                Does anything bring them on?
                  IF SPECIFIC SITUATION DESCRIBED:
                        Do they only occur in these situations, or have these attacks also sometimes come on from out of the blue, or in situations where you did not expect them?

Do you worry a lot about having more of them?
    IF YES: How long would it take before you would stop worrying that another attack would occur?

What are you afraid might happen from these anxiety attacks?
    (Do you worry a lot that you might have a heart attack?
      Are you often worried that you might go crazy or lose control?
        IF YES TO EITHER: How long have you worried about that?)

Have you changed your behavior or routine since these attacks began?

A panic attack refers to a discrete period of intense fear or discomfort, in which at least four of the following symptoms developed abruptly and reached a peak within 10 minutes.

Think of the last bad attack you had. When was it? Where were you at the time? I'm going to ask you about some symptoms you may have experienced during that attack. Did you...

1) ...feel your heart racing, pounding, fluttering, or skipping beats?
2) ...sweat?
3) ...tremble or shake?
4) ...have trouble catching your breath, or feel like you were being smothered?
5) ...feel like you were choking?
6) ...have chest pain, pressure, tightness, or discomfort?
7) ...feel nauseated, sick to your stomach, or like you might have diarrhea?
8) ...feel dizzy, light-headed, unsteady, or like you might faint?
9) ...feel like things around you were unreal, like you were in a dream, like parts of your body were unreal or detached from you, or like you were outside of yourself, watching?
10) ...fear you were going crazy or might lose control?
11) ...fear you might die?
12) ...feel numb or tingling in your fingers or feet?
13) ...have hot flashes or chills?

During a bad attack, how long does it usually take from the time it begins until you have most of the symptoms like [SYMPTOMS NOTED ABOVE]?
   (IF UNCLEAR OR GREATER THAN TEN MINUTES):
   Would most of the symptoms ever come on quickly, within ten minutes after the attack began?

(B) <u>Exclude</u> the diagnosis if the symptoms are due to the direct physiological effects of a substance (e.g., a drug of abuse, a medication) or a general medical condition (e.g., hyperthyroidism).

(C) <u>Exclude</u> the diagnosis if the anxiety is better accounted for by another mental disorder, such as obsessive-compulsive disorder, posttraumatic stress disorder, separation anxiety disorder, specific phobia, or social phobia.

AGORAPHOBIA

> Inclusion: A, B
> Exclusion: C

Diagnostic Note: Agoraphobia can be diagnosed with or without a history of panic disorder. See pages 40-41 for panic disorder questions.

(A) Anxiety about being in places or situations from which escape might be difficult (or embarrassing) or in which help might not be available in the event of having an unexpected or situationally predisposed panic attack or panic-like symptoms. Agoraphobic fears typically involve characteristic clusters of situations that include being outside the home alone; being in a crowd or standing in a line; being on a bridge; and traveling in a bus, train, or car. NOTE: Consider the diagnosis of specific phobia if the avoidance is limited to one or only a few specific situations, or social phobia if the avoidance is limited to social situations.

Some people have very strong fears of being in certain places or in certain situations. Do any of the following make you feel very fearful, anxious, or nervous?

  a) Being away from home alone.
  b) Being in crowded places like a movie theater, supermarket, shopping mall, church, restaurant, etc.
  c) Standing in long lines.
  d) Being on a bridge or in a tunnel.
  e) Traveling in a bus, train, or plane.
  f) Driving or riding in a car.
  g) Being home alone.
  h) Being in wide open spaces like a park.
  i) Being in a closed in space (e.g., small rooms, elevators)
  IF YES TO ANY OF ABOVE:
  I know it may be difficult to describe, but what is it about [PHOBIA] that worries you?
  What do you think might happen to you?
  What are you afraid of?

(B)	The situations are avoided (e.g., travel is restricted), or else endured with marked distress or with anxiety about having a panic attack or panic-like symptoms, or require the presence of a companion.

> To what degree do you avoid [PHOBIA]?
> **IF NO AVOIDANCE:**
> > So what do you do, how do you cope?
> > Does having someone with you help?
> > Do you [PHOBIA] only when you're with someone?
> > Do you [PHOBIA] alone?
> > > **IF YES:** How bad does the anxiety get?
> > > What are you anxious about?

(C)	<u>Exclude</u> the diagnosis if the anxiety or phobic avoidance is better accounted for by another mental disorder, such as obsessive-compulsive disorder (e.g., avoidance of contamination); post-traumatic stress disorder (e.g., avoidance of stimuli associated with a severe stressor); separation anxiety disorder (e.g., avoidance of leaving parents); social phobia (e.g., avoidance limited to social situations because of fear of embarrassment); or specific phobia (e.g., avoidance limited to a single situation like elevators).

SOCIAL PHOBIA

> Inclusion: A-E
> Exclusion: F, G

(A) **A marked and persistent fear of one or more social or performance situations in which the person is exposed to unfamiliar people or to possible scrutiny by others. The individual fears that he or she will act in a way (or show anxiety symptoms) that will be humiliating or embarrassing.**

Some people have very strong fears of being watched or evaluated by others. Do you worry that you might do or say something that would embarrass you in front of others, or that other people might think badly of you?

Let me ask about some specific situations. Do any of the following make you feel more fearful, anxious, or nervous than most people?

a) Eating in front of others.
b) Writing in front of others.
c) Public speaking.
d) Saying something when in a group of people.
e) Asking a question when in a group of people.
f) Urinating in public restrooms.
g) Business meetings.
h) Parties.
   IF YES TO ANY: Do you think you are much more anxious than other people?

I know it may be difficult to describe, but what is it about [PHOBIA] that worries you (e.g., choking when eating; hand trembling with writing; being unable to urinate; not being able to complete a lecture, speech, or presentation)?

(B) **Exposure to the feared social situation almost invariably provokes anxiety, which may take the form of a situationally bound or situationally predisposed panic attack.**

Whenever you [PHOBIA] do you immediately get anxious or nervous?
   IF YES: What is that like?
      Do you have a panic attack?
   IF NO, OR THERE IS COMPLETE AVOIDANCE OF PHOBIC STIMULUS: What about in the past?

(C)	**The person recognizes that the fear is excessive or unreasonable.**

> Do you think you are more afraid and worried about [PHOBIA] than you should be?
> **IF NO:** You <u>really</u> don't believe that you worry too much about [PHOBIA]?
> > **IF NO:** Then why do you think other people aren't as concerned about/worried by [PHOBIA]?

(D)	**The feared social or performance situations are avoided, or else endured with intense anxiety or distress.**

> To what degree to you avoid [PHOBIA]?
> **IF NO AVOIDANCE:** How bad does the anxiety get when you [PHOBIA]? Do you have a panic attack?

(E)	**The avoidance, anxious anticipation, or distress in the feared social or performance situation(s) interferes significantly with the person's normal routine, occupational (academic) functioning, or social activities or relationships, or there is marked distress about having the phobia.**

> What problems in your life has the avoidance/fear of [PHOBIA] caused?
> Has it caused job (or school) problems like getting fired or failure to get promoted?
> What about marital problems?
> What about interfering with friendships?
> What about affecting leisure time activities?
> How much does it bother you that you have this fear of [PHOBIA]?

(F)	<u>Exclude</u> the diagnosis if the fear or avoidance is due to the direct physiological effects of a substance (e.g., drugs of abuse, medication) or a general medical condition, or is better accounted for by panic disorder with or without agoraphobia, specific phobia, separation anxiety disorder, body dysmorphic disorder, a pervasive developmental disorder, or schizoid personality disorder.

(G)	<u>Exclude</u> the diagnosis if the fear is related to another psychiatric or physical disorder (e.g., fear of a panic attack, stuttering, Parkinsonian trembling, anorexic or bulimic abnormal eating behavior).

SPECIFIC PHOBIA (SIMPLE PHOBIA)

| Inclusion: A-E |
| Exclusion: F |

(A) Marked and persistent fear that is excessive or unreasonable, cued by the presence or anticipation of a specific object or situation (e.g., flying, heights, animals, receiving an injection, seeing blood).

Some people have very strong fears of certain objects or situations. Do any of the following make you feel very fearful or nervous?

a) Heights
b) Being near household pets like cats or dogs
c) Spiders, bugs, snakes, mice, or bats
d) Flying
e) Seeing blood
f) Being in water (e.g., swimming pools, lakes)
g) Storms
h) Receiving an injection
   IF YES TO ANY: Do you think you are more anxious than other people?

NOTE: Do not include fears related to agoraphobia or social phobia.

(B) Exposure to the phobic stimulus almost invariably provokes an immediate anxiety response, which may take the form of a situationally bound or situationally predisposed panic attack.

Whenever you [PHOBIA] do you immediately get anxious or nervous?
   IF YES: What is that like?
      Do you have a panic attack?
   IF NO, OR THERE IS COMPLETE AVOIDANCE OF PHOBIC STIMULUS: What about in the past?

(C) The person recognizes that the fear is excessive or unreasonable.

Do you think you are more afraid and worried about [PHOBIA] than you should be?
   IF NO: You <u>really</u> don't believe that you worry too much about [PHOBIA]?
      IF NO: Then, why do you think other people aren't as concerned about/worried by [PHOBIA]?

Specific Phobia (Simple Phobia) 47

(D)	The phobic situation(s) is avoided, or else endured with intense anxiety or distress.

To what degree do you avoid [PHOBIA]?
  IF NO AVOIDANCE:
    How bad does the anxiety get when you [PHOBIA]?
    How upset do you get when you [PHOBIA]?

(E)	The avoidance, anxious anticipation, or distress in the feared situation(s) interferes significantly with the person's normal routine, occupational (academic) functioning, or social activities or relationships, or there is marked distress about having the phobia.

What problems in your life has the avoidance/fear of [PHOBIA] caused? Has it interfered with your routine?
What about job (or school) problems?
What about marital problems?
What about interfering with friendships?
What about affecting leisure time activities (e.g., outings, vacations)?
How much does it bother you that you have this fear of [PHOBIA]?

(F)	<u>Exclude</u> the diagnosis if the anxiety, panic attacks, or phobic avoidance associated with the specific object or situation are better accounted for by another mental disorder, such as obsessive-compulsive disorder (e.g., fear of contamination); posttraumatic stress disorder (e.g., avoidance of stimuli associated with a severe stressor); separation anxiety disorder (e.g., avoidance of school); social phobia (e.g., avoidance of social situations because of fear of embarrassment); panic disorder, or agoraphobia.

GENERALIZED ANXIETY DISORDER

> Inclusion: A, B, at least 3 from C, E
> Exclusion: D, F

(A) **Excessive anxiety and worry (apprehensive expectation), occurring more days than not for at least six months, about a number of events or activities (such as work or school performance).**

During the past several months, have you been frequently worried or anxious about a number of events or activities in your daily life?
> **IF YES:** What have you worried about?
>> Do people say you worry about these things too much?
>> Do you think you do?
>> Do you think your anxiety is unrealistic or excessive?
>> Do you worry that something bad is going to happen to you, or to someone close to you?
>> How often do you worry about these things? (On more days than not?)
>> For how long? (Has it been at least six months?)

(B) **The person finds it difficult to control the worry.**

Is it hard for you to control or stop your worrying?

(C) **The anxiety and worry are associated with at least three of the following six symptoms (with at least some symptoms present for more days than not for the past six months).**

Now I'm going to ask you about physical symptoms that often go along with anxiety and nervousness. During the past 6 months, when you are feeling nervous or tense, do you often...

1) ...feel restless, fidgety, jittery, keyed up, on edge, or have difficulty sitting still?
2) ...get tired very easily?
3) ...have problems concentrating, or does your "mind go blank?"
4) ...feel irritable?
5) ...feel tension, aches, or soreness in your muscles?
6) ...have problems falling asleep or staying asleep?

How often do you have these physical symptoms? (On more days than not?)

(D)	<u>Exclude</u> the diagnosis if the focus of the anxiety and worry are confined to experiencing features of another Axis I disorder, such as anxiety or worry about having a panic attack (as in panic disorder), being embarrassed in public (as in social phobia), being contaminated (as in obsessive-compulsive disorder), gaining weight (as in anorexia nervosa), having multiple physical complaints (as in somatization disorder), or having a serious illness (as in hypochondriasis), and the anxiety and worry do not occur exclusively during posttraumatic stress disorder.

(E)	The anxiety, worry, or physical symptoms cause clinically significant distress or impairment in social, occupational, or other important areas of functioning.

What effect has the anxiety, worry, and [SYMPTOMS FROM C] had on your life?
Does it bother you a lot that you feel this way?
Has it affected your job (school)?....marriage?.... relationship with friends?....social life?...leisure activities?
   IF YES: In what way?

Does it interfere with or keep you from completing your daily routine and chores?

(F)	<u>Exclude</u> the diagnosis if the symptoms are due to the direct effects of a substance (e.g., a drug of abuse, a medication) or a general medical condition (e.g., hyperthyroidism), or are present only during the course of a mood disorder, a psychotic disorder, or a pervasive developmental disorder.

POSTTRAUMATIC STRESS DISORDER

> Inclusion: A1, A2, at least 1 from B, 3 from C, 2 from D, E, F
> Exclusion: None

(A1) **The person has been exposed to a traumatic event in which he/she experienced, witnessed, or was confronted with an event or events that involved actual or threatened death or serious injury, or a threat to the physical integrity of oneself or others.**

Have you ever seen or experienced a traumatic event in which your life was actually in danger, or you thought your life was in danger?
  IF YES: What happened?

Have you ever witnessed an event in which someone else's life seemed to be in danger?
  IF YES: What happened?

What about traumatic events in which you or someone else were seriously injured, or could have been seriously injured?
  IF YES: What happened?

(A2) **The person's response to the traumatic event involved intense fear, helplessness, or horror.**

How did you react when you [TRAUMA]?
(Were you frightened or horrified?)
(Did you feel helpless and out of control?)

B. **The traumatic event is persistently reexperienced in at least one of the following ways:**

(B1) **Recurrent and intrusive distressing recollections of the event, including images, thoughts, or perceptions.**

Do memories about the [TRAUMA] still bother you?
Do you see images of the trauma?
  IF YES TO EITHER: Tell me about them. How frequent are they? Do you try to put them out of you head, but sometimes can't?

(B2) **Recurrent distressing dreams of the event.**

What about dreams of the [TRAUMA]? (Describe)

(B3) Acting or feeling as if the traumatic event were recurring (includes a sense of reliving the experience, illusions, hallucinations, and dissociative flashback episodes, including those that occur on awakening or when intoxicated).

Some people who experience such terrible events sometimes have flashbacks where they relive the event, and they may even act or feel as though the event is happening again, even though it isn't. Has this happened to you?
IF YES: Describe.
IF NO: Have you ever had hallucinations of the episode? (Have you heard voices or seen visions from the [TRAUMA])?

(B4) Intense psychological distress at exposure to internal or external cues that symbolize or resemble an aspect of the traumatic event.

Are there things that remind you of the [TRAUMA] that get you upset?
IF YES: Describe.
IF NO: Do you feel bad on the anniversary of the [TRAUMA]?

(B5) Physiological reactivity upon exposure to internal or external cues that symbolize or resemble an aspect of the traumatic event.

Do reminders of the [TRAUMA] make you tremble, break out into a sweat, hyperventilate, or have a racing heart?

C. Persistent avoidance of stimuli associated with the trauma and numbing of general responsiveness (not present before the trauma), as indicated by at least three of the following:

(C1) Efforts to avoid thoughts, feelings, or conversations associated with the trauma.

Do you try to block out thoughts or feelings related to the [TRAUMA]? Do you avoid talking about it?

(C2) Efforts to avoid activities, places, or people that arouse recollections of the trauma.

Do you try to avoid activities, situations, or places that remind you of the [TRAUMA]? **IF YES:** Like what?
Do you avoid people who remind you of it?

(C3) Inability to recall an important aspect of the trauma.

Are there some aspects of the [TRAUMA] that you can't recall?
IF YES: Like what?

(C4) Markedly diminished interest or participation in significant activities.

Have you noticed that since the [TRAUMA] you've lost interest in some things you used to enjoy? **IF YES:** Like what?

Are there any activities you no longer participate in since it occurred? **IF YES:** Like what?

(C5) Feeling of detachment or estrangement from others.

Do you frequently feel like you don't fit in with the people around you? That is, you're with them physically but you feel distant and cutoff from them.

(C6) Restricted range of affect (e.g., unable to have loving feelings).

Does it seem like you've lost the ability to feel certain emotions?
IF YES: Like what?
Do you feel emotionally numb?
(Has it seemed like you no longer have strong feelings about anything, or you can't feel love anymore?)

(C7) Sense of a foreshortened future (e.g., does not expect to have a career, marriage, children, or a normal life span).

Has the [TRAUMA] changed how you feel about the future?

Have you given up on some goals that you used to have for yourself? **IF YES:** Like what?

After a traumatic event some people feel different about things they've always wanted such as a career, marriage, having kids, living a long life. Did the trauma affect you in any way like this?
IF YES: In what way?

D.	Persistent symptoms of increased arousal (not present before the trauma), as indicated by at least two of the following:

(D1)	Difficulty falling or staying asleep.

Since the [TRAUMA] have you had problems sleeping?

(D2)	Irritability or outbursts of anger.

Have you been more irritable or lost your temper more easily?

(D3)	Difficulty concentrating.

Since the [TRAUMA] have you had problems concentrating?
   IF YES: In what areas?

(D4)	Hypervigilance.

Since the [TRAUMA] have you been on the alert, always keeping your guard up with an eye out for possible trouble?

(D5)	Exaggerated startle response.

Have you been kind of jumpy and easily startled by everyday, ordinary noises and movement?

(E)	Duration of the disturbance (symptoms in Criteria B, C, and D) is more than one month.

For how long have you been bothered by (SYMPTOMS IN B-D)?

(F)	The disturbance causes clinically significant distress or impairment in social, occupational, or other important areas of functioning.

What effect has this trauma had on your life?

Do you often feel extremely upset or distressed because of it?

Has it affected your job (school)?....marriage?....relationship with friends?....social life?...leisure activities? **IF YES:** In what way?

Has it interfered with or kept you from completing your daily routine and chores?

ACUTE STRESS DISORDER

> Inclusion: A1, A2, at least 3 from B, C-G
> Exclusion: H

(A1) The person has been exposed to a traumatic event in which he/she experienced, witnessed, or was confronted with an event or events that involved actual or threatened death or serious injury, or a threat to the physical integrity of oneself or others.

Have you ever seen or experienced a traumatic event in which your life was actually in danger, or you thought your life was in danger?
  IF YES: What happened?

Have you ever witnessed an event in which someone else's life seemed to be in danger?
  IF YES: What happened?

What about traumatic events in which you or someone else were seriously injured, or could have been seriously injured?
  IF YES: What happened?

(A2) The person's response to the traumatic event involved intense fear, helplessness, or horror.

How did you react when you [TRAUMA]?
(Were you frightened or horrified?)
(Did you feel helpless and out of control?)

B. Either while experiencing or after experiencing the distressing event, the individual has at least three of the following dissociative symptoms:

(B1) A subjective sense of numbing, detachment, or absence of emotional responsiveness.

What was your emotional reaction while it was happening?
What about after it happened?
Either while the [TRAUMA] happened, or afterwards, did you feel emotionally numb, or like you no longer had strong feelings about anything? Did you feel distant and cutoff from people?

(B2)	A reduction in awareness of his or her surroundings (e.g., "being in a daze").

Did you feel like you were "in a daze?"

Did it seem like you were less aware of everything else going on around you?

(B3)	Derealization.

While it was happening, or afterwards, did it seem like things were unreal, or like everything was a dream?
Did things around you seem somehow strange, or changed in shape or size?
   IF YES TO EITHER: Describe what that was like.

(B4)	Depersonalization.

Did it seem like your body or some part of your body was somehow changed, not real, or detached from you?

Did you feel like you were watching yourself from outside your body?

(B5)	Dissociative amnesia (i.e., inability to recall an important aspect of the trauma).

After the [TRAUMA] did you have a brief blackout, and forget some important aspect of the event?

(C)	The traumatic event is persistently reexperienced in at least one of the following ways: recurrent images, thoughts, dreams, illusions, flashback episodes, or a sense of reliving the experience; or distress on exposure to reminders of the traumatic event.

Do memories about the [TRAUMA] still bother you?
Do you see images of the trauma?
   IF YES TO EITHER: Tell me about them. How frequent are they? Do you try to put them out of you head, but sometimes can't?

What about dreams of the [TRAUMA]? (Describe)

Some people who experience such terrible events sometimes have flashbacks where they relive the event. They may either act or feel as though the event is happening again, even though it isn't. Has this happened to you?
  IF YES: Describe.
  IF NO: Have you ever had hallucinations of the episode? (Have you heard voices or seen visions from the [TRAUMA])?

Are there things that remind you of the [TRAUMA] that get you upset?
  IF YES: Describe.
  IF NO: Do you feel bad on the anniversary of the [TRAUMA]?

Do reminders of the [TRAUMA] make you tremble, break out into a sweat, hyperventilate, or have a racing heart?

(D) **Marked avoidance of stimuli that arouse recollections of the trauma (e.g., thoughts, feelings, conversations, activities, places or people).**

Do you try to block out thoughts or feelings related to the [TRAUMA]? Do you avoid talking about it?

Do you try to avoid activities, situations, or places that remind you of the [TRAUMA]? **IF YES:** Like what?

Do you avoid people who remind you of it?

(E) **Marked symptoms of anxiety or increased arousal (e.g., difficulty sleeping, irritability, poor concentration, hypervigilance, exaggerated startle response, and motor restlessness).**

Since the [TRAUMA] have you had problems sleeping?

Have you been more irritable or lost your temper more easily?

Since the [TRAUMA] have you had problems concentrating?
  IF YES: In what areas?

Since the [TRAUMA] have you been on the alert, always keeping your guard up with an eye out for possible trouble?

Have you been kind of jumpy and easily startled by everyday, ordinary noises and movement?

Have you felt fidgety or restless?

(F)	The disturbance causes clinically significant distress or impairment in social, occupational, or other important areas of functioning or impairs the individual's ability to pursue some necessary task, such as obtaining necessary assistance or mobilizing personal resources by telling family members about the traumatic experience.

What effect has this trauma had on your life?

Do you often feel extremely upset or distressed because of it?

Has it effected your job (school)?....marriage?....relationship with friends?....social life? **IF YES:** In what way?

Has it interfered with or kept you from completing your daily routine and chores?

Were you able to tell your family what happened?
    IF YES: How hard was it to go to them?

ASK FOLLOWING QUESTIONS IF APPROPRIATE AND NECESSARY:

Were you able to get the medical help you needed?
Did you go to the police?
    IF NO TO EITHER: What kept you from doing that?

(G)	The disturbance lasts for a minimum of two days and a maximum of four weeks and occurs within four weeks of the traumatic event.

For how long have you been bothered by [SYMPTOMS IN B-E]?

How soon after the trauma happened did the symptoms like [SYMPTOMS IN B-E] begin?

(H)	<u>Exclude</u> the diagnosis if the symptoms are due to the direct effects of a substance (e.g., a drug of abuse, a medication) or a general medical condition, are better accounted for by brief psychotic disorder, and are not merely an exacerbation of a preexisting Axis I or Axis II disorder.

OBSESSIVE-COMPULSIVE DISORDER

> Inclusion: A1-A4 for obsessions or
> A1-A2 for compulsions
> B and C for either
> Exclusion: D, E

A. OBSESSIONS - A1-A4 are all required

(A1) Recurrent and persistent thoughts, impulses, or images that are experienced, at some time during the disturbance, as intrusive and inappropriate and cause marked anxiety and distress.

Some people are bothered by recurrent thoughts or impulses that seem inappropriate or do not make sense, but they keep repeating over and over and are difficult to get out of their mind. (For example, intrusive, repeated thoughts that you might hurt or kill someone you love even though you didn't want to; that someone you love is hurt; that you will yell obscenities in public; that you are contaminated by germs or dirt; or that you just hit someone while driving.) Has anything like this been a problem for you?
  IF YES: Describe what it's like.
    How often does it happen?
    How do you feel when you have these thoughts?

What about intrusive, frequent, repeated images?
  IF YES: Tell me about it.
    How often does it happen?
    How do you feel when you have these images?

(A2) The thoughts, impulses, or images are not simply excessive worries about real-life problems.

(A3) The person attempts to ignore or suppress such thoughts, impulses or images, or to neutralize them with some other thought or action.

What do you do to deal with this?

Do you try to ignore or get rid of these thoughts/images and put them out of your mind?

Do you tell yourself things or imagine certain other images in order to neutralize or counteract the unpleasant thought/image?

(A4) The person recognizes that the obsessional thoughts, impulses, or images are a product of his or her own mind (not imposed from without as in thought insertion).

Are these your own thoughts, or do you believe they are put into your head by someone, or some force or power from the outside?
   IF OUTSIDE: Tell me about how that happens.

COMPULSIONS - A1 and A2 are both required

(A1) Repetitive behaviors (e.g., hand washing, ordering, checking), or mental acts (e.g., praying, counting, repeating words silently) that the person feels driven to perform in response to an obsession, or according to rules that must be applied rigidly.

Some people are bothered by having to do something over and over that they can't resist when they try. For example, they wash their hands repeatedly, check whether the door is locked or the stove is turned off, or count things excessively. Have you had any difficulties like this?
   IF YES: Like what?
          Describe what it's like.

Do you have any rituals that you always have to do in a particular order, and if the order is wrong you have to start all over from the beginning? **IF YES:** Like what?

(A2) The behaviors or mental acts are aimed at preventing or reducing distress or preventing some dreaded event or situation; however, these behaviors or mental acts either are not connected in a realistic way with what they are designed to neutralize or prevent or are clearly excessive.

If you do not [COMPULSION], do you get very anxious or tense?
   IF NO: So, why do you do it?

What do you think might happen if you didn't [COMPULSION]?

Criteria B-E are the same for both obsessions and compulsions.

(B)	**At some point during the course of the disorder, the person has recognized that the obsessions and compulsions are excessive or unreasonable.**

> Does the [OBSESSION/COMPULSION] seem unreasonable or excessive, but you still feel compelled to do it?
> **IF NO:** Did you <u>ever</u> think the [OBSESSION/COMPULSION] was unreasonable or excessive?
> **IF NO:** Did other people think so?
> **IF YES:** What did they say?
> Do you think they're wrong?

(C)	**The obsessions or compulsions cause marked distress, are time-consuming (take more than an hour a day), or significantly interfere with the person's normal routine, occupational (or academic) functioning, or usual social activities or relationships.**

> Does it bother you a lot that you have the [OBSESSION/COMPULSION]?
>
> What effect has it had on your life?
>
> Has it affected your job (school)?....marriage?....relationship with friends?....social life?....leisure activities?
> **IF YES:** In what way?
>
> Does it keep you from completing your daily routine and chores?
>
> How much time a day do you spend [OBSESSION/COMPULSION]?

(D)	<u>Exclude</u> the diagnosis if another axis I disorder is present, and the content of the obsessions or compulsions is restricted to it (e.g., preoccupation with food in the presence of an eating disorder; hair pulling in the presence of trichotillomania; concern with appearance in the presence of body dysmorphic disorder; preoccupation with having a serious illness in the presence of hypochondriasis).

(E)	<u>Exclude</u> the diagnosis if it is due to the direct physiological effect of a substance (e.g., a drug of abuse, a medication) or a general medical condition.

SOMATIZATION DISORDER

> Inclusion: A, B1-B4
> Exclusion: C

(A) A history of many physical complaints beginning before age 30 years that occur over a period of several years and result in treatment being sought or significant impairment in social, occupational or other important areas of functioning.

How's your physical health been most of your life?
Do you get sick more than most people?
> **IF EVIDENCE OF CHRONIC POOR HEALTH:**
> What's been the matter?
> Would you say you've been sickly most of your life?
> Do you usually go to the doctor when you're feeling sick?
> About how many times a year do you go to the doctor? ER?
> What effect has your poor physical health had on your life?
> Has it effected your job (school)?....marriage?....relationship with friends?....social life? **IF YES:** In what way?

B. For a symptom to be counted towards the diagnosis, the symptom must not be fully explained by a known general medical condition or by the direct effect of a substance, or the resulting complaints or impairment from a general medical condition are in excess of what would be expected from the history, physical examination, or laboratory findings.

Follow-up questions for positive responses:
> Did you go to the doctor for that?
> What did the doctor say was wrong?
> What problems did the [SYMPTOM] cause you?

(B1) Four pain symptoms:

Have you had a lot of trouble with...
- (1) ...abdominal or belly pain (other than when menstruating)?
- (2) ...pain in your arms or legs?
- (3) ...back pain?
- (4) ...pain in your joints?
- (5) ...pain when you urinate?
- (6) ...headaches?
- (7) chest pain?
- (8) pain during sex?
- (9) excessively painful menstrual periods?
- (10) pain anywhere else?

(B2) Two gastrointestinal symptoms (other than pain):

Have you had a lot of trouble with...
- (1) ...vomiting (other than during pregnancy)?
- (2) ...nausea without vomiting (other than motion sickness)?
- (3) ...excess gas or bloating of your stomach?
- (4) ...diarrhea?
- (5) ...foods you cannot eat because they make you ill?

(B3) One sexual symptom (other than pain):

(1) In general, has your sex life been important to you, or could you have gotten along as well without it?

FOR MEN ONLY:
(2) Has there ever been a time when you had trouble having an erection?
Have you ever had difficulty ejaculating?
IF YES: What caused the problem?

FOR WOMEN ONLY:
(3) Have your periods usually been pretty regular or irregular?
IF IRREGULAR: Are they more irregular than most women?

(4) Do you usually bleed very heavy?
IF YES: More than most women?

(5) **IF NOT ALREADY KNOWN:** Have you ever been pregnant?
IF YES: What were your pregnancies like?
Did you ever have a lot of problems with vomiting?
IF YES: Did you vomit throughout any of your pregnancies?

***DIAGNOSTIC REMINDER: For a symptom to be counted towards the diagnosis, the symptom must meet the general criteria for B described on page 61.

(B4) One pseudoneurologic symptom:

Did you ever...
- (1) ...have a period of amnesia--like a blackout or a lost period of time where you couldn't remember what happened?
- (2) ...have difficulty swallowing?
- (3) ...have shortness of breath when not exerting yourself?
- (4) ...lose your voice?
- (5) ...go complete deaf for a short while?
- (6) ...have double vision (not due to needing glasses)?
- (7) ...go totally blind for a short while?
- (8) ...faint?
- (9) ...have a seizure or convulsion?
- (10) ...have problems with numbness? **IF YES:** Where?
- (11) ...have trouble walking?
- (12) ...have problems with your balance or coordination?
- (13) ...have problems with muscle weakness so that you couldn't lift or move things like normal, or paralysis when you were completely unable to move a part of your body?
- (14) ...have difficulty urinating?

(C) <u>Exclude</u> the diagnosis if the symptoms are intentionally produced or feigned (as in factitious disorder or malingering).

HYPOCHONDRIASIS

> Inclusion: A, B, D, E
> Exclusion: C, F

(A) Preoccupation with fears of having, or the idea that one has, a serious disease based on the person's misinterpretation of bodily symptoms.

> How is your physical health?
> (Do you have any physical problems?)
>
> Do you worry a lot about your physical health?
> **IF YES:** What do you think might be wrong?
> How hard is it to get your mind off of this?
>
> Do you often worry about the possibility that you have some type of serious illness?
> **IF YES:**
> What symptoms do you have that make you worry about this?
> What do you think might be wrong?
> How hard is it to get your mind off of this?

(B) The preoccupation persists despite appropriate medical evaluation and reassurance.

> Did you see a doctor about these problems?
> **IF YES:** What kind of evaluation did he/she do?
>
> What did your medical doctor say was the matter?
>
> Did he/she have a diagnosis?
>
> **IF DOCTOR SAID THERE WAS NO EVIDENCE OF SERIOUS MEDICAL PROBLEM:**
> How did that make you feel?
> Did you believe him/her?
> (Is it hard for you to believe your doctor when he/she tells you there is nothing to worry about?)
> Did you stop thinking about [PHYSICAL PROBLEM]?
> **IF YES:** After awhile, do you start thinking that you might be ill again?

(C)	<u>Exclude</u> the diagnosis if the belief is of delusional intensity (as in delusional disorder, somatic type), and is not restricted to a circumscribed concern about appearance (as in body dysmorphic disorder).

> Is it possible that you don't have [DISEASE]?
> **IF NO:** Are you sure?
> Then why do you think the doctor hasn't diagnosed it?

(D)	The preoccupation causes clinically significant distress or impairment in social, occupational, or other important areas of functioning.

> What effect has your worrying (or thinking) about having [PHYSICAL ILLNESS] had on your life?
>
> How upsetting has it been?
>
> Does it bother you a lot that you have these concerns?
>
> Has this affected your job (school)?....marriage?....relationship with friends?....social life?....leisure activities?
> **IF YES:** In what way?
>
> Does it interfere with or keep you from completing your daily routine and chores?

(E)	The duration of the disturbance is at least six months.

> For how long have you been worrying or thinking about this?

(F)	<u>Exclude</u> the diagnosis if the preoccupation is better accounted for by generalized anxiety disorder, obsessive-compulsive disorder, panic disorder, a major depressive episode, separation anxiety, or another somatoform disorder.

BODY DYSMORPHIC DISORDER

> Inclusion: A, B
> Exclusion: C

(A) **Preoccupation with an imagined defect in appearance. If a slight physical anomaly is present, the person's concern is markedly excessive.**

Do you often think there is something wrong with the way you look?
Do you often think you look gross, disfigured, or ugly?
  IF YES TO EITHER: To what are you referring?
  How much do you think about this?
  How hard is it to get your mind off of this?
  Have you talked to your friends or family about this?
    IF YES: What do they say?
    Do they try to convince you that you are wrong and that you don't look the way you think you do?

(B) **The preoccupation causes clinically significant distress or impairment in social, occupational, or other important areas of functioning.**

What difficulties in your life has your concern about your appearance caused?
Has it caused problems in your job (school)?....marriage?
....relationships with friends or family?....social life?....leisure activities?
  IF YES TO ANY: What kind of problems?
  IF NO TO ALL: Have you been socially withdrawn because of your concern about your appearance?

Have you seen a doctor to fix your [PHYSICAL DEFECT]?
  IF YES: What did the doctor recommend or do?

Did you ever have surgery?

(C) <u>Exclude</u> **the diagnosis if the preoccupation is better accounted for by another mental disorder (e.g., dissatisfaction with body shape and size in anorexia nervosa).**

TRICHOTILLOMANIA

> Inclusion: A, B, C, E
> Exclusion: D

(A) Recurrent pulling out of one's hair resulting in noticeable hair loss.

Do you frequently pull out your hair from your head, eyebrows, or other parts of your body?
> **IF YES:** From what parts of your body do you pull your hair?
> Do you pull out enough so that it is noticeable (to others)?

(B) An increasing sense of tension immediately before pulling out the hair or when attempting to resist the behavior.

Do you feel compelled to pull out your hair?
> **IF YES:** Describe what that's like.

Do you get somewhat tense or anxious immediately before you pull?

Do you get tense or anxious when you try to resist pulling?

(C) Pleasure, gratification, or relief when pulling out the hair.

How do you feel immediately after you pull?

Is there any sense of pleasure?

What about tension release or relief?

(D) <u>Exclude</u> the diagnosis if it is better accounted for by another mental disorder or it is due to a general medical condition (e.g., a dermatological disorder.)

(E) The disturbance causes clinically significant distress or impairment in social, occupational, or other important areas of functioning.

What effect has the hair pulling had on your life?

How upsetting is it? Does it bother you a lot that you do this?

Has this affected your job (school)?....marriage?....relationship with friends?...social life?...leisure activities? **IF YES:** In what way?

Does it interfere with or keep you from completing your daily routine and chores?

ATTENTION-DEFICIT/HYPERACTIVITY DISORDER

> Inclusion: A1 or A2, B, C, D
> Exclusion: E

A. EITHER (A1) OR (A2):

A1. Inattention: At least six of the following symptoms of inattention have persisted for at least six months to a degree that is maladaptive and inconsistent with developmental level:

****
NOTE: For each symptom you must inquire whether it is present more than most boys/girls the child's age.
****

(1) Often fails to give close attention to details or makes careless mistakes in schoolwork, work, or other activities.

Some kids have problems paying close attention to things, and because of this they make a lot of careless mistakes in their schoolwork. Is this something you do?
   IF YES: Does it happen a lot?
            Does it affect your grades?
What about things around the house. Do you often make careless mistakes when doing chores around the house?
   IF YES: Examples.

(2) Often has difficulty sustaining attention in tasks or play activities.

Some kids have a hard time staying on track or keeping their mind on the things they are doing because they can't pay attention to one thing for a long time. Is it hard for you to pay attention to only one thing for a long time?

Is it hard for you to stick with one thing, even when it's fun?

Is it hard to focus on a test or an assignment that lasts an entire period?

Is it hard to play a game that lasts a long time like Monopoly?
   IF YES TO ANY: Do you frequently have difficulty focusing on one thing for a long time?
                    Does your poor attention span cause you difficulties?

(3)	**Often does not seem to listen when spoken to directly.**

How good are you at listening to what your parents or teachers say to you?

Do your teachers say that you don't listen when they talk to you?

Do they have to ask you the same thing over and over before you listen?

What about with your parents. Do they often have to repeat what they say to you? Do they sometimes say you "must be deaf?"
    IF EVIDENCE OF POOR LISTENING:
        How often does this happen?

(4)	**Often does not follow through on instructions and fails to finish schoolwork, chores, or duties in the workplace (not due to oppositional behavior or failure to understand instructions).**

Some kids have difficulty finishing things. Is that true of you?

Is it hard to finish your homework or schoolwork, even when you know how to do it?
    IF YES: Is it hard to stick with it, or do you stop doing it because
          you don't like doing it?

What about things around the house. Do you start doing them and leave in the middle?
    IF YES: Do you do that a lot?
          Is it hard to stick with it, or do you stop doing it because
          you don't like doing it?

(5)	**Often has difficulty organizing tasks and activities.**

Is it hard for you to be organized?
    IF YES: Tell me about that.

Is it difficult to plan and organize your schoolwork?
    IF YES: What happens?

Do you need your mom's or dad's help getting organized to do school projects?
    IF YES: What would happen?

(6)	**Often avoids, dislikes, or is reluctant to engage in tasks that require sustained mental effort (such as schoolwork or homework).**

Some kids really hate doing schoolwork or homework because it's hard for them to concentrate on it for a long time. Are you like that?

(7)	**Often loses things necessary for tasks or activities (e.g., school assignments, pencils, books, tools, or toys).**

Do you lose things a lot?

At school do you frequently forget your pen or pencil, or leave your books or homework in the wrong place?

What about toys, keys, and money? Do you lose or misplace them a lot?

(8)	**Is often easily distracted by extraneous stimuli.**

Some kids find it hard to keep their mind on the things they are doing, even when it's fun. Is it hard for you to keep playing a game when you hear something in the next room?
How easy is it for someone to get your attention when you're watching your favorite TV program?
    IF DISTRACTED: So, is it hard for you to focus on one activity for a long time?
                        Does this happen a lot?
                        Does it happen at school? At home, too?

(9)	**Is often forgetful in daily activities.**

Are you very forgetful?
What types of things do you forget to do?
Do you often forget to do things like brushing your teeth, washing your hands, changing your underwear?
    IF YES: Is this forgetfulness, or is it that you don't like doing these things?

Attention-Deficit/Hyperactivity Disorder

A2. <u>Hyperactivity-Impulsivity</u>: At least six of the following symptoms of hyperactivity-impulsivity have persisted for at least six months to a degree that is maladaptive and inconsistent with developmental level:

---

(1) Often fidgets with hands or feet or squirms in seat.

Is it hard for you to sit still?

Is it hard to sit still while watching television, playing a game, or doing homework, or while you're sitting in class at school?

Has anyone ever said that you can't seem to sit still, or that it seems like you have "ants in your pants?"

---

(2) Often leaves seat in classroom or in other situations in which remaining seated is expected.

Is it hard for you to stay in your seat in school?

Do you get out of your seat a lot when you're not supposed to?
   IF YES: Tell me about that.
          Have you gotten into trouble for it?

Do you stay in your chair during all of breakfast or all of dinner, at home or at a restaurant, or do you get up a lot?

---

(3) Often runs about or climbs excessively in situations in which it is inappropriate (in adolescents or adults, may be limited to subjective feelings of restlessness).

Do you run around the house or climb on furniture a lot?

Do you climb on desks or other things in school?

Do you jump down the stairs or run down the halls?
   IF YES TO ANY: Tell me about it.
                  Do your teachers/parents often have to tell you to stop running around so much?
                  Do you get into trouble for this? Does it happen a lot?

(4)	Often has difficulty playing or engaging in leisure activities quietly.

Do your parents frequently tell you to quiet down when you play?
Are you noisier than other kids your age?
Is this a problem at school?

(5)	Is often "on the go" or acts as if "driven by a motor".

Are you often on the go, doing something?
Are you more active than other kids your age?
Does it feel like there's a motor inside you that keeps you going all the time?

(6)	Often talks excessively.

Do you talk a lot? **IF YES:** More than other kids?

Do your parents or teachers say that you're a chatterbox because you never stop talking?

(7)	Often blurts out answers before questions have been completed.

When your teachers ask questions in class do you tend to answer the question out loud before the teacher has a chance to finish asking it?
   IF YES: How often does this happen?
            Has your teacher spoken to you or your parents about this?

(8)	Often has difficulty awaiting turn.

For some kids it is hard for them to wait their turn when playing games. Is this hard for you?
   IF YES: What problems does this cause?

Is it hard for you to wait on line in stores, or going to movies, or other activities where you have to wait on line?
Do you often try to cut in line?

When you eat with your family is it hard for you to wait to get served?
   IF YES: Do other people get angry with you because of this?

(9)	**Often interrupts or intrudes on others (e.g., butts into conversations or games).**

> Do your parents get angry at you because you butt into their conversations?
>
> Do your parents get angry because you interrupt them while they're on the phone?
> **IF YES:** Does this happen a lot?
>
> Do other kids tell you to leave them alone so they could do their work?
>
> Do you butt into other kids games before they ask you to play?

(B)	**Some hyperactive-impulsive or inattentive symptoms that caused impairment were present before age seven years.**

> **IF TIME COURSE NOT ALREADY ESTABLISHED:**
> How old were you when you began (BEHAVIORS NOTED ABOVE)? What problems did this cause?

(C)	**Some impairment from the symptoms is present in two or more settings (e.g., at school [or work] and at home).**

(D)	**There must be clear evidence of clinically significant impairment in social, academic, or occupational functioning.**

> **IF IMPAIRMENT NOT ALREADY ESTABLISHED:**
> What problems do (BEHAVIORS NOTED ABOVE) cause?
> Do (BEHAVIORS) bother your parents a lot?
> Does it cause school problems?
> What problems does it cause with other kids?
> Did you see a doctor or school counselor or anyone else like that?
> Did you take medication for (BEHAVIORS)?

(E)	<u>Exclude</u> **the diagnosis if it occurs exclusively during the course of a pervasive developmental disorder, schizophrenia or other psychotic disorder, and is not better accounted for by another mental disorder (e.g., a mood disorder, anxiety disorder, dissociative disorder, or a personality disorder).**

CONDUCT DISORDER

> Inclusion: At least 3 from A, B
> Exclusion: C

Now I'm going to ask you about some different types of behaviors that sometimes get children and teenagers into trouble.

A. A repetitive and persistent pattern of behavior in which the basic rights of others or major age-appropriate societal norms or rules are violated, as manifested by the presence of at least three of the following criteria in the past twelve months, with at least one criterion present in the past six months.

AGGRESSION TO PEOPLE AND ANIMALS

(A1) Often bullies, threatens, or intimidates others.

Do you pick on other kids?
   IF YES: How often?
       Do you pick on kids that are younger or smaller than you? Describe.

Are you a bully?

Do you ever threaten other kids so they will buy you things, give you money, or do other things for you?
   IF YES: How often? Describe.

(A2) Often initiates physical fights.

Do you get into many fights? (More than other kids?)
   IF YES: How often?
       How often do you start the fights?

(A3) Has used a weapon that can cause serious physical harm to others (e.g., a bat, brick, broken bottle, knife, gun).

Have you ever used a weapon in a fight?
   IF YES: What did you use?
       For what reason?
       How often did that happen?

(A4) Has been physically cruel to people.

Have you hurt people physically?
IF YES: What did you do to them? For what reason?

(A5) Has been physically cruel to animals.

Have you ever hurt, tortured, or killed an animal?
IF YES: What did you do?

Do you have a pet?
IF YES: Did you ever deliberately hurt it?

(A6) Has stolen while confronting a victim (e.g., mugging, purse snatching, extortion, armed robbery).

Have you ever taken things from people like snatching a purse, jewelry, or chains?

Have you ever held anyone up, or robbed a store?

Have you ever threatened anyone if they didn't give you money?

(A7) Has forced someone into sexual activity.

Have you ever forced anyone to have sex with you?

Were you ever part of a group or gang that forced someone to have sex against his/her will?
IF YES: Tell me about that.

DESTRUCTION OF PROPERTY

(A8) Has deliberately engaged in fire setting with the intention of causing serious damage.

Have you ever set things on fire?
IF YES: Why?

(A9) Has deliberately destroyed others' property (other than by fire setting).

Have you ever damaged someone's property by breaking windows, spraying graffiti on walls, or other things like that?
IF YES: What did you do?

DECEITFULNESS OR THEFT

(A10) Has broken into someone else's house, building, or car.

> Have you ever broken into anyone's house, a store, building or car?
> **IF YES:** For what reason?
> Did you do it alone or with someone?

(A11) Often lies to obtain goods or favors or to avoid obligations (i.e., "cons" others).

> Sometimes kids don't tell the truth; they make up stories. Do you make up stories that aren't truthful?
> **IF YES:** What kinds of things do you make up stories about?
>
> Do you tell a lot of lies?
> **IF YES:** Do you lie a lot or a little?
>
> Do you often lie to get things that you wanted?
>
> Do you often lie to avoid chores or other responsibilities?

(A12) Has stolen items of nontrivial value without confronting a victim (e.g., shoplifting, burglary, forgery).

> How often have you stolen from stores, your parents, or other people?
> **IF YES:** What did you steal?
> What's the most you've stolen?
>
> Did you ever get caught stealing?
> **IF YES:** What happened?
>
> Did you ever pick anyone's pocket, write a forged check, or use a credit card without permission?

SERIOUS VIOLATIONS OF RULES

(A13) Often stays out all night despite parental prohibitions, beginning before 13 years of age.

> Do you argue with your parents about how late you could stay out at night?
> Do you often stay out later than they said you could?
> Did you ever stay out all night?
> **IF YES:** How old were you when you first began doing this?

(A14) Has run away from home overnight at least twice while living in parental or parental surrogate home (or once without returning for a lengthy period).

> Did you ever run away from home overnight?
> **IF YES:** How often?
> How long did you stay away?

(A15) Is often truant from school, beginning before 13 years of age.

> Have you ever played hooky or skipped school?
> **IF YES:** How many times did you do it?
> Did you get into trouble for it?
> How old were you?
> How old were you when you started to skip school?

(B) The disturbance in behavior causes significant impairment in social, academic, or occupational functioning.

> You mentioned that you (BEHAVIORS ACKNOWLEDGED ABOVE).
>
> What problems did this cause?
>
> Does it cause problems at school? (Expulsion? Suspension?)
>
> How does it affect your friendships, or family life?
>
> Have you ever seen a doctor, counselor, or anyone else for this?

(C) <u>Exclude</u> the diagnosis if age 18 or older and meets criteria for antisocial personality disorder.

OPPOSITIONAL DEFIANT DISORDER

> Inclusion: At least 4 from A, B
> Exclusion: C, D

***

NOTE: For each symptom you must inquire whether it is present more than most boys/girls the child's age.

***

A. A pattern of negativistic, hostile, and defiant behavior lasting at least six months, during which time at least four of the following are present:

(A1) Often loses temper.

What happens when you get angry and mad?

Does this happen a lot?

Do you have a bad temper?
   IF YES: Tell me about that.

Is your temper so big that you can't stop it?

Do you have temper tantrums?
   IF YES: What causes them?
             How often do you have them?

(A2) Often argues with adults.

Do you frequently argue with your parents or teachers?
   IF YES: About what?
            Do you always find something to argue about?

(A3) Often actively defies or refuses to comply with adults' requests or rules.

Is it hard for you to follow rules?

Do you think that most rules are pretty stupid?
   IF YES: Tell me about that.

Do you like to break rules on purpose?

Do you often say no when your parents or teachers ask you to do something?
   IF YES: Like what?

(A4) Often deliberately annoys people.

> Do you like to do things that annoy or bother other people?
> **IF YES:** Like what?
> How often do you do things like that?

(A5) Often blames others for his or her mistakes or misbehavior.

> Is it hard for you to admit that you are wrong when you make a mistake?
>
> Do you blame other people for your mistakes?
>
> Do you blame other people when you misbehave or get into trouble?

(A6) Is often touchy or easily annoyed by others.

> What do your parents or teachers do that bothers you?
>
> Is it easy for others to annoy you?

(A7) Is often angry and resentful.

> Do you feel angry a lot of the time?
> **IF YES:** Why is that?
>
> Does it often bother you that other people boss you around or tell you what to do?
> **IF YES:** Tell me about that.
>
> Do you think that you are treated unfairly?
> **IF YES:** By whom?
> In what way?

(A8) Is often spiteful or vindictive.

> **IF YES TO ANY QUESTION IN #7:**
> What do you do about _____?
> How do you get back at _____?

Oppositional Defiant Disorder

(B)	The disturbance in behavior causes significant impairment in social, academic, or occupational functioning.

You mentioned that you (BEHAVIORS ACKNOWLEDGED ABOVE).

What problems did this cause?

Does it cause problems at school? (Suspension? Transfer?)

Has it caused you to lose friends?

What about problems at home?

Have you ever seen a doctor, counselor, or anyone else for this?

(C)	<u>Exclude</u> the diagnosis if behaviors occur exclusively during the course of a psychotic or mood disorder.

(D)	<u>Exclude</u> the diagnosis if person meets criteria for conduct disorder or, if age 18 or older, meets criteria for antisocial personality disorder.

SEPARATION ANXIETY DISORDER

> Inclusion: At least 3 from A, B, C, D
> Exclusion: E

A. Developmentally inappropriate and excessive anxiety concerning separation from home or from those to whom the child is attached, as evidenced by at least three of the following:

(A1) Persistent and excessive worry about losing, or possible harm befalling, major attachment figures.

(MAF = Major Attachment Figure, i.e., mother, father, etc.)

Do you worry a lot that something bad will happen to your MAF?

Do you worry a lot that they will go away and never come back?

Do you often get scared that they will get hurt or die?
   IF YES TO ANY: Why are you scared about that?
   For how long have you been worrying about this?

(A2) Persistent and excessive worry that an untoward event will lead to separation from a major attachment figure (e.g., getting lost or being kidnapped).

Do you get scared a lot about getting lost when you leave the house with your MAF?

Do you get scared that your MAF will leave you and not come back?

Do you get scared that you or your MAF will be kidnapped and you'd never see them again?
   IF YES TO ANY: How often do you worry that _____?
   For how long have you been worrying about this?

(A3)	Persistent reluctance or refusal to go to school or elsewhere because of fear of separation.

Do you get any nervous or scared feelings about going to school?
    IF YES: Tell me about that.

When you first started going to school was it hard for you to go because you didn't want to be away from your MAF?
    IF YES: Did they have to drag you to school?
            Did you refuse to go?

(A4)	Persistently and excessively fearful or reluctant to be alone or without major attachment figures at home or without significant adults in other settings.

Is it scary for you to be alone at home?

Do you feel upset if an adult isn't always with you?
    IF YES TO EITHER: How old were you when you started to feel this way?

(A5)	Persistent reluctance or refusal to go to sleep without being near a major attachment figure or sleep away from home.

Do you sleep alone or with your parents?
Are you afraid of going to sleep alone?
Does your MAF have to stay nearby or with you till you fall asleep?
Is it hard to sleep when your MAF isn't around?
Do you sometimes not go to sleep until your MAF is in the home?

Are you allowed to sleep at someone else's house?
    IF YES: Have you ever been invited to stay at someone's house?
            IF YES: Did you go?
                    IF NO: Why not?
                    IF YES: How was it being away from your MAF?

(A6)	Repeated nightmares involving the theme of separation.

Do you have a lot of scary dreams or nightmares?
    IF YES: What are they about?
           (Do you have any about being separated from you MAF - like being kidnapped or your MAF going away?)

(A7)	**Repeated complaints of physical symptoms (such as headaches, stomachaches, nausea, or vomiting) when separation from major attachment figure occurs or is anticipated.**

Do you get physically sick when you are not with your MAF?

Do you often get sick before you go to school in the morning?

Do you get physically sick thinking that your MAF is going somewhere without you?
   IF YES TO ANY: What part of your body gets sick?
   How often does this happen?

(A8)	**Recurrent excessive distress when separation from home or major attachment figure occurs or is anticipated.**

Do you get upset or nervous when you are away from home?

Do you get upset when you see your MAF going out without you?

Do you get upset just thinking that your MAF is going somewhere without you?
   IF YES TO ANY: What do you do? (Call home? Go home early? Cry? Scream? Have a temper tantrum?)

(B)	**Duration of the disturbance is at least four weeks.**

IF NOT CLEAR FROM ABOVE INFORMATION:

For how long have you (SYMPTOMS NOTED ABOVE)?

(C)	**Onset before age 18.**

(D)	**The disturbance causes clinically significant distress or impairment in social, academic (occupational), or other important areas of functioning.**

What problems have the (BEHAVIORS NOTED ABOVE) caused?

Have your grades suffered or have you missed a lot of school?

Has it affected the number of friends you have?

Have you ever see a doctor, counselor, or anyone else for this?

(E)	<u>Exclude</u> the diagnosis if the symptoms occur exclusively during the course of a pervasive developmental disorder, schizophrenia, or other psychotic disorder, and in adults and adolescents, is not better accounted for by panic disorder with agoraphobia.

FUNCTIONAL CAUSES OF DEPRESSION AND ANXIETY

DEPRESSION AND ANXIETY DUE TO DRUGS, MEDICATION, AND MEDICAL ILLNESS

Lists of medications and physical illnesses that have been found to be associated with anxiety and depression symptoms and syndromes are presented on the next three pages. These lists are not exhaustive (for example, more than 200 medications have been implicated in causing depression), but instead represent the most commonly described "organic" causes or mimics of anxiety and depression.

Obviously, patients with anxiety or depression are not usually worked up to rule out all of these potential causes. Findings from the history and physical examination will determine which laboratory and diagnostic tests to order. The level of the physician's intervention will depend on the suspected cause of the psychiatric symptoms.

In many instances treatment of the underlying illness will eliminate the anxiety or depression (e.g., endocrine disorders). If the course of psychopathology parallels the initiation of a medication known to sometimes cause anxiety or depression, then changing to an alternative medication may be effective (e.g., switching from reserpine or a beta blocker to another antihypertensive). Sometimes it will be necessary to simply wait and monitor the symptoms of depression or anxiety over a few weeks to avoid treating psychiatric symptoms unnecessarily (e.g., withdrawal from alcohol, cocaine, amphetamines). Finally, pharmacologic intervention will often be necessary, even in cases where the psychiatric symptoms seem to be an understandable reaction to the negative consequences of a severe medical illness (e.g., depressive syndrome associated with a cerebrovascular accident).

COMMONLY USED MEDICATIONS ASSOCIATED WITH DEPRESSION

Antihypertensives

Clonidine
Guanethidine
Hydralazine
Methyldopa
Beta blockers
Reserpine
Thiazides
Spironolactone

Sedatives

Alcohol
Barbiturates
Benzodiazepines
Chloral Hydrate

Steroids

Corticosteroids
Oral Contraceptives
Prednisone

Dopamine Agonists

Amantadine
Bromocriptine
Levodopa

Anticonvulsants

Phenytoin
Carbemazepine

Analgesics

Ibuprofen
Indomethacin
Opiates

H^2 Blockers

Cimetidine
Ranitidine

Stimulant Withdrawal

Amphetamines
Cocaine

Other

Metoclopramide
Tamoxifen

MEDICAL ILLNESSES ASSOCIATED WITH DEPRESSION

Endocrine

Addison's disease
Cushing's syndrome
Hypo- and Hyperadrenocorticism
Hypo- and Hyperthyroidism
Hypo- and Hyperparathyroidism
Carcinoid syndrome
Pancreatic carcinoma
Premenstrual syndrome
Postpartum syndrome
Hypoglycemia
Hyperaldosteronism

Immunologic

Rheumatoid arthritis
Systemic lupus erythematosus
Temporal arteritis
Sjogren's syndrome

Infection

HIV
Mononucleosis

Metabolic

Acute intermittent porphyria
Pernicious anemia
Wilson's disease

Neurologic

Cerebral syphilis
Encephalitis
Epilepsy
Huntington's disease
Hydrocephalus
Migraines
Multiple sclerosis
Cerebral neoplasm
Cerebrovascular disease
Narcolepsy
Parkinson's disease
Stroke (especially left sided)

Withdrawal States

Alcohol
Cocaine

Vitamin Deficiencies

Folate
Vitamin B^{12}
Niacin
Vitamin C
Thiamine

Systemic

Anemia
Renal failure
Systemic neoplasm

MEDICAL ILLNESSES AND COMMONLY USED DRUGS ASSOCIATED WITH ANXIETY

Endocrine

Addison's disease
Cushing's syndrome
Hypo- and Hyperadrenocorticism
Hypo- and Hyperthyroidism
Hypo- and Hyperparathyroidism
Carcinoid syndrome
Pancreatic carcinoma
Pheochromocytoma
Hypoglycemia

Cardiovascular

Anemia
Cardiac arrhythmia
Congestive heart failure
Hypovolemia
Mitral valve prolapse
Myocardial infarction
Angina

Respiratory

Asthma
Hypoxia
Pneumonia
Pneumothorax
Pulmonary edema
Pulmonary embolus
Postoperative atelectasis

Immunologic

Polyarteritis nodosa
Rheumatoid arthritis
Systemic lupus erythematosis
Temporal arteritis

Infection

HIV
Mononucleosis
Viral hepatitis

Metabolic

Acidosis
Acute intermittent porphyria
Pernicious anemia
Wilson's disease

Neurologic

Cerebral syphilis
Encephalitis
Epilepsy (especially temporal lobe)
Huntington's disease
Migraines
Multiple sclerosis
Meniere's disease
Postconcussive syndrome
Cerebrovascular disease

Withdrawal States

Alcohol
Narcotics
Caffeine
Nicotine
Sedative-hypnotics

Drugs

Amphetamines
Sympathomimetics
Penicillin
Sulfonamides
Cocaine
Caffeine
Indomethacin
Appetite suppressants

MINI-MENTAL STATE EXAMINATION

The Mini-Mental State Examination (MMSE, Folstein et al, 1975) is the most widely used screening evaluation for cognitive impairment. The MMSE has been used to screen for dementia and delirium, grossly quantify the degree of cognitive impairment, and serially measure cognitive changes over time. It should be emphasized that the MMSE is only a screening measure, and it should not be used as the sole criterion for diagnosing dementia.

The MMSE is reprinted on the next two pages. Scores range from 0-30, and values of 23 or less suggest the presence of cognitive impairment. Some authorities recommend that three levels of cognitive impairment be delineated: 24-30 = no cognitive impairment; 18-23 = mild cognitive impairment; and 0-17 = severe cognitive impairment. MMSE scores are correlated with years of education, and the established cutoff points are probably not valid if the patient has less than a ninth grade education.

The MMSE has been reprinted with permission from: Folstein MF, Folstein SE, and McHugh PR. "Mini-mental State:" A practical method for grading the cognitive states of patients for the clinician. *Journal of Psychiatric Research*, 1975, *12*: 189-198.

MINI-MENTAL STATE EXAM (Folstein)

Now I'm going to ask you some questions to test your concentration and memory.

ORIENTATION TO TIME
( ) What year is this? [1 point]
( ) What season of the year is it? [1 point]
( ) What is the month and date? [1 point for each]
( ) What day of the week is it? [1 point]

ORIENTATION TO PLACE
( ) What is the name of this place? [1 point]
( ) What floor are we on? [1 point]
( ) What city and state are we in? [1 point for each]
( ) What county is this? [1 point]

IMMEDIATE RECALL
( ) I am going to say 3 objects. After I say them, I want you to repeat them. They are: "Apple" "Table" "Penny." Now you say them. Remember what they are because I'm going to ask you to name them again in a few minutes. [1 point for each]
(Interviewer: Repeat until all 3 are learned.)

ATTENTION (either item)
( ) a) Subtract 7 from 100, then subtract 7 from the answer you get and keep subtracting 7 until I tell you to stop. [1 point for each correct answer, maximum 5 points]
b) Spell the word "world" backwards. [1 point for each correct letter, maximum 5 points]

DELAYED RECALL
( ) What are the 3 words I asked you to remember? [1 for each]

NAMING
( ) Show patient wrist watch and pen and ask to name them. [1 point for each]

REPETITION
( ) Repeat the following sentence exactly as I say it. "No ifs, ands, or buts." [1 point]

3 STAGE COMMAND
( ) Now I want to see how well you can follow instructions. I'm going to give you a piece of paper. Take it in your right hand, use both hands to fold it in half, and then put it on the floor. [1 point for each command, maximum 3 points]

READING
( ) Show patient page 91 and ask patient to read what it says at the top of the page silently, to him/herself, and then do what it says. [1 point]

COPYING
( ) Give patient clean sheet of paper and ask him/her to copy the design printed on page 91. [1 point]

WRITING
( ) On same sheet of paper, ask patient to write a complete sentence. [1 point]

( ) **Total** (Maximum score = 30)

CLOSE YOUR EYES

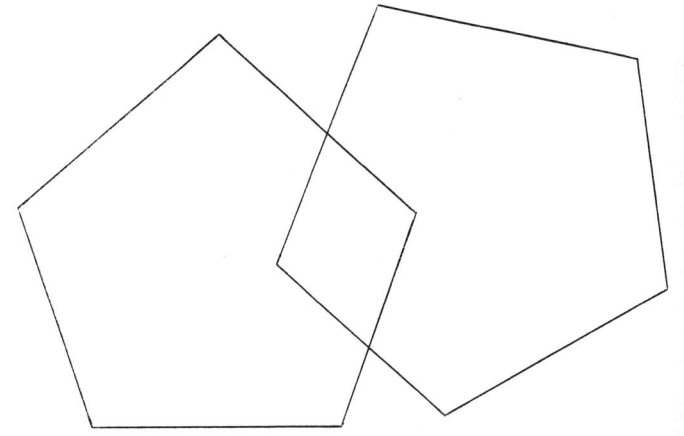

BRIEF PSYCHOSOCIAL HISTORY

Now, I'd like to ask you some questions about your childhood and some other areas of your life.

CHILDHOOD
Where were you born and raised?
  (When did you move?) (Why did you move?)
Were your parents married?
Did your mother have problems with the pregnancy or delivery?
Did you reach your developmental milestones, like walking, talking, potty training, on time?

With whom did you live while you were growing up?
Who did you feel closest to?
Who in the family was affectionate to you?
How did you get along with [PERSONS RAISING PATIENT]?

Who made the rules and enforced discipline?
Were the family rules pretty clear and consistently applied?
Do you think the rules were fair?
How often did you get punished?
How did they usually discipline you?
Did they ever spank or hit you?
    IF YES: Did they ever leave bruises when they hit you?
        Did you ever have to see a doctor?

Did you see violence in the family?
Did anyone sexually abuse you?
    IF YES: What happened?
        How often did it occur?
        How much did this upset you at the time?
        What about now?

At what age did you begin school?
Did you go to regular or special classes?
    IF SPECIAL CLASSES: Why?
How did you do in school? (What were your grades?)
Did you ever repeat a grade?
What was the last grade you completed?
Were you involved in school activities? **IF YES:** Like what?
What did you do after you graduated (or dropped out)?

What was your personality like as a child?
Did you have many friends as a child?
    (Did you have any really close friends? Best friends?)
Were you more of a leader or a follower?

PARENTHOOD
Do you have any children?
IF YES: How many? What are their ages and sexes?
How do you get along with them?

FRIENDSHIPS AND MARRIAGE
Do you have many friends now?
(Any close friends, that is, someone you can really trust with secrets?)
(Do you tend to keep friends for a long time?)

Have you ever been married?
IF YES: How many times?
How would you describe your marriage(s)?
IF DIVORCED: Why did you divorce?
IF NO: How come you never got married?

Almost all couples argue or fight, and I'd like to know a little bit about what happens when you and your partner have disagreements. Do you or your partner ever get pushed, grabbed, or hit during these times? What about throwing things?
IF YES: Describe the most recent (or serious) time that this happened.
How often does something like this happen?
Have you ever had to go to a doctor because of injuries received during a fight?
IF NO: Did this ever happen in prior relationships? (Tell me about it.)
Are you ever afraid that you will be physically hurt during or after an argument with your (SPOUSE, BOY/GIRLFRIEND)?

OCCUPATION
Are you employed?
IF YES: What kind of work do you do?
How long have you worked there? Do you like it?
What other jobs have you had? Why did you leave?
What's the longest job you've ever had?
IF NO: When was the last time you worked? What happened?
What kind of job was it?
What other jobs have you had?
What's the longest job you've ever had?

LIVING SITUATION
Where do you live?
Do you live in an apartment? A house?
How long have you been living there?
(Where did you previously live?)
(Why did you move?) (Have you moved much?)
(Have you ever not had a place to stay? What did you do?)
With whom do you live?

CURRENT PSYCHOSOCIAL FUNCTIONING

___
Employment
___

Do you work?
IF YES:
> What kind of work do you do?
> How many hours per week do you work?
> Did you miss any time from work during the past week?
> > **IF YES:** How much time did you miss?
> > > For what reason?
>
> Did you have any problems on the job during the past week?
> > **IF YES:** Like what?
>
> Does anyone evaluate your performance at work? **IF YES:** Who?
> Does anyone (else) give you feedback on your performance?
> **IF YES:** Who?
> > **IF YES TO EITHER:**
> > > What do they look at to determine whether you're doing a good job?
> > > What kind of evaluations have you gotten?
> > > What do <u>you</u> look at to determine if you're doing a good job?
> > > How well did you do your job during the past week?
> > > Could you give me some examples?
> >
> > **IF NO TO BOTH:**
> > > What do <u>you</u> look at to determine if you're doing a good job?
> > > How well did you do your job during the past week?
> > > Could you give me some examples?
>
> **IF NOT ALREADY CLEAR FROM ABOVE:**
> > In what way did your (PATIENT DESCRIPTION OF HEALTH PROBLEM) effect your job during the past week?
> > Because of your (HEALTH PROBLEM), were there things you didn't get done at work?
> > > **IF YES:** Like what?
> >
> > Did your (HEALTH PROBLEM) cause problems concentrating at work?
> > Did you work as efficiently as usual?
> > > **IF NO:** Describe that for me.

IF NO: Why didn't you work this past week?

Household work

What responsibilities do you have in your household?
Do you do any cleaning?
Laundry?
Cooking?
Shopping?
House repairs or yard work?
Take care of any kids or older or disabled family members?
Run errands?
Is there anything else that you do to keep your household running?

During this past week how well have you been keeping up with your household responsibilities?

Are there any things you usually do that you didn't get done this past week?
   IF YES: What kept you from (TASK)?
                Were there days you didn't get anything done?
                    IF YES: How many days were like that?

Did you have any difficulty doing your household chores?
   IF YES: Like what?

How would you rate your performance of household chores for the past week?
Can you give me some examples?

IF NOT ALREADY CLEAR FROM ABOVE:
   In what way did your (HEALTH PROBLEM) affect your (SPECIFIC CHORES)?
   Because of (HEALTH PROBLEM), were there things you didn't get done?
      IF YES: Like what?
   Were there things you didn't do as well as usual?
      IF YES: Like what?

Schoolwork

Do you go to school or take any classes?
    IF YES: Are you a full-time student?
               IF NO: How many classes do you take?

ASK THE FOLLOWING IF AT LEAST A HALF-TIME STUDENT

Did you miss or skip any classes this past week?
    IF YES: How many?
                For what reason?

Were you given any assignments, homework, or tests this past week?
    IF YES: How did you do?
               IF UNSURE: How do you think you did? (How do you
                                    usually do?)

How have your study habits been this past week?

IF EVIDENCE OF IMPAIRED FUNCTIONING:
Were there days you didn't get anything done? That is, you couldn't
go to classes or you couldn't do any homework or studying?
    IF YES: How many days were like that?

IF NOT ALREADY CLEAR FROM ABOVE:
How did your (HEALTH PROBLEM) specifically affect your schoolwork
this past week?
Did your (HEALTH PROBLEM) cause problems concentrating?
Did you work as efficiently as usual?
    IF NO: Describe that for me.

Relationships with husband, wife, boyfriend, girlfriend, or lover

Are you married?
> **IF YES:** How would you describe your marriage?
> How close a relationship do you and your spouse usually have?
> How were things this past week?
> Did you have any arguments or disagreements this past week?
>> **IF YES:** How often did you argue?
>> For how long did you stay angry at each other?
>> Were you able to work out your problems?

> **IF NO:** Do you have a boyfriend or girlfriend or lover?
>> **IF YES:** How long have you been going with him/her?
>> Do you live together?
>> How close a relationship do you and your partner usually have?
>> How have you gotten along this past week?
>> Did you have any arguments or disagreements this past week?
>>> **IF YES:** How often did you argue?
>>> For how long did you stay angry at each other?
>>> Were you able to work out your problems?

IF NOT ALREADY CLEAR FROM ABOVE:
How did your (HEALTH PROBLEM) affect your relationship?
Did it affect your closeness?
Have you been more withdrawn?
Did you argue more or less?

Relationships with other family members

Who is in your immediate family? Your extended family? Do you have in-laws? Grandparents? Grandchildren? Any other family?

Are your parents still alive?
    IF YES: Are you close?
                How do you get along with them?
                Did you see or speak to them this past week?
                How have you gotten along with them this past week?
                Did you have any arguments or disagreements this past week?
                      IF YES: How often did you argue?
                                    For how long did you stay angry at each other?

Do you have any brothers or sisters?
    IF YES: Are you close?
                How do you get along with them?
                Did you see or speak to them this past week?
                How have you gotten along with them this past week?
                Did you have any arguments or disagreements this past week?
                      IF YES: How often did you argue?
                                    For how long did you stay angry at each other?

Do you have any children?
    IF YES: Are you close?
                How old are they?
                Did you see or speak to them this past week?
                How have you gotten along with them this past week?
                Did you have any arguments or disagreements this past week?
                      IF YES: How often did you argue?
                                    For how long did you stay angry at each other?

Are there family members that you avoid seeing because of serious problems or trouble getting along?

IF NOT ALREADY CLEAR:
    How did your (HEALTH PROBLEM) affect your relationships with your family?
    Did it effect your closeness with anyone?
    Have you been more withdrawn?
    Did you argue more or less with anyone?

Relationships with friends

Not counting your family members, do you have any close friends you can confide in about a personal matter?
    IF YES: How many close friends do you have?
                 How often do you usually see or speak to them?
                 What about this past week?
                 How have you been getting along with them over the past week?
                 Any arguments or disagreements?
                 How strong are the ties between you?

    IF NO: How many people do you know that you wouldn't necessarily confide in, but whom you would consider friends?
        IF ONE OR MORE:
            How often do you usually see or speak to them?
            What about this past week?
            How have you been getting along with your friends over the past week?
            Any arguments or disagreements?
            How strong are the ties between you?

IF NOT ALREADY CLEAR:
    How did your (HEALTH PROBLEM) effect your relationships with your friends?
    Did it effect your closeness with anyone?
    Have you been more withdrawn?
    Did you argue more or less with anyone because of your (HEALTH PROBLEM)?

Recreation

What kinds of leisure or recreational activities do you enjoy?
Do you have any hobbies?
(Are there any activities [outside of work] that you do regularly or occasionally?)
What did you do for fun this past week?

What about: reading?
　　　　　　watching or playing sports?
　　　　　　participating in community groups?
　　　　　　exercising?
　　　　　　gardening?
　　　　　　going to the movies, plays or concerts?
　　　　　　crafts?
　　　　　　watching television?
　　　　　　listening to or playing music?
　　　　　　going to church, synagogue or temple?
　　　　　　hobbies?
　　　　　　parties?

How often did you (ACTIVITY MENTIONED ABOVE)?

How much did you enjoy (ACTIVITY)?

How much did your (HEALTH PROBLEM) affect your participation in leisure, recreational and fun activities?

How much did your (HEALTH PROBLEM) affect your enjoyment of the things you did?

General satisfaction with life

We've reviewed several areas of your life - work, housework, relationships with family and friends, and leisure. The last thing I'd like to ask you about is your level of satisfaction with your life. Considering all the different areas of your life, how satisfied overall have you felt about your life during the past week?
- **IF GENERALLY SATISFIED:**
    - Are you satisfied with all areas of your life?
        - **IF NO:** Which areas are you dissatisfied with?
            - How dissatisfied are you?
        - **IF YES:** Any dissatisfaction in any areas?
            - **IF YES:** Which ones?
                - How dissatisfied are you?
- **IF GENERALLY DISSATISFIED:**
    - Are you dissatisfied with all areas of your life?
        - **IF NO:** Which areas are you satisfied with?
            - How satisfied are you?
        - **IF YES:** Any satisfaction in any area?
            - **IF YES:** Which ones?
                - How satisfied are you?

ORDERING INFORMATION

Title: Diagnosing DSM-IV Psychiatric Disorders in Primary Care Settings
ISBN: 0-9633821-4-4

PRICE LIST

# copies	Cost
1-4	$9.00 (plus $3.50 Shipping & Handling [S/H]) = $12.50/copy
5-24	$9.00/copy (S/H included)
25-100 [15% off]	$7.75/copy (S/H included)
> 100	Call for price quote

All orders will be shipped via UPS. Prepayment by check or money order is necessary.

Payable to: Psych Products Press

Mailing address: Psych Products Press
P.O. Box 228
East Greenwich, RI 02818

Phone: (401) 885-6746

# of copies: _____

Shipping address: _____